We Don't Talk About That:

A Cultural Analysis of the Miscarriage Experience Through the Words of Women who Lived It

By: Grace Gould

Artwork By: Alex Krales

Edited By: Dr. Pamela Stone, Dr. Marlene Fried

I would like to thank many different souls for the creation of this project.

To Lisa, Jennifer, Cindy, Jenn, Susan, Jenni, Amy, Lexi, Malissa, Shannon, Amber, Kirsten and all of the women who contacted me to be interviewed: I cannot thank you enough for offering to share your story.

To Carroll from SHARE, PLSP and Jenn: thank you so much for connecting me to women who wanted to tell their stories.

To Marlene, Pam and Richard: Thank you for teaching me, for letting me take all of your classes, and for caring about what I do. You were incredible mentors for the road less traveled.

To Grammy, Ghee, Mom, Keith, Cameron, Cartie, Rashka, Kelby, Luke, Mattyhead, and Hampshire friends: Thanks for getting me through this project.

To Alex Krales: Thank you for your wonderful artwork.

To Cherry Jones, Dr. Davis, and all of the individuals who helped me realize my love for reproductive health: Thank you.

Table of Contents

Introduction

I decided to embark on this project while sitting in traffic on the Jackie Robinson parkway during a warm evening in September. Its origins, however, began years before. My awareness with miscarriage started the day I was twelve years old and sitting in the break room of the OB/GYN where my grandmother worked. I don't remember why I had been brought along, and I don't remember how long I had been there. But I do recall that I had been sitting alone a long time and would gladly continue existing in such a state if it meant I never had to know why.

At some point, my mother walked into the room. I don't remember her telling me and I don't remember what was said. What I have memorized is her image. My mother had seemed so foreign to me when she became pregnant. That was a state I assumed would never exist, and the change in her body unsettled me. She was wearing black, and I remember looking at her almost from a distance and recognizing that her body would only be in this form for a while longer. What it signified was a lost possibility that would soon catch up to itself. I remember looking at her stomach; she had finally begun to show in the past month. I was very confused. Something that had officially made its notification in the world couldn't fail.

When I was twelve years old, my mother had a miscarriage at five months as a result of a chromosomal abnormality. After being told the news in the break room, nothing more was said. The only awareness I had that the pregnancy did not magically disappear was a paper sitting on my mother's makeup table a week later that mentioned sticks, seaweed, and bleeding. Once I read the word "intercourse" I stopped reading and never mentioned any of it. This horrible thing was done, it would never happen again, and that was that.

My second awareness of miscarriage occurred on a plane a year later when my mother turned to me and told me that she was pregnant. I smiled, but I didn't believe her. I did not want another pregnancy. I did not want a sibling. And I did not want to sit in that break room again. I didn't have to. She lost the pregnancy at 12 weeks while eating at a restaurant in North Carolina. We were on vacation with our family, so I was sent off with the aunts and cousins and did not see her much. I only learned it had ended on the way home in the car when my mother mentioned to my stepfather how much blood there was; she kept bleeding and it didn't seem like it xwould ever stop. That was all I ever heard. My mother got divorced and remarried her college sweetheart; I went to high school and grew up. Everything that had happened blended into a past chapter that was closed.

I moved to college in Massachusetts, became interested in reproductive rights, and focused on pregnancy, birth and abortion. I attended births in the United States and the Philippines. I wrote a birth guide and studied how race and oppression affect pregnancy. I was consumed by women's health. My mother would talk about pregnancy, and she would talk about birth. She refused to talk about abortion or any possibilities of pregnancy not working out.

Close to the end of my second year in college, my father suddenly died. The contrast of my studies and my life was too much. I now understood a grief that very few if any around me did, and the isolation of my sadness pushed me away from the happy birth movement I had been so enthusiastic about. I returned home that summer to regain my feet and threw myself into my work. I had gotten a job as an assistant at the OB/GYN where my grandmother worked. What a summer. I saw everything; pregnancies, contraception, diseases, infections, babies, and postpartum. The most significant experience I had, however, was realizing what had happened while I was waiting in the break room all those years ago. Not all the pregnancies worked out. Perhaps it was the proximity I had to grief at that moment, but a loss always meant a long drive home. I had reached my saturation point; this was something I did not want to think about. So I didn't.

I went back to college for my third year and continued my work. Increasingly, what I studied seemed to fit into what I can only describe as a reproductive life spectrum. Every reproductive occurrence in a woman's life fits somewhere along this, and each influences the other. The problem was that I felt I was missing something. I had studied birth and abortion, life and death. But what was in between? In the spring and the midst of my confusion over what to do my final thesis (Division III) about, my friend mentioned that she had experienced a miscarriage. That was it.

5

I walked home, called my mother, and started to unbury what had been hiding for years. First, however, I had to get through my summer internship working with a doctor at Mount Sinai in New York City. The barrage of patients, stories, terminations, operations, research, blood and humidity completely wore me down. I finished the summer having shifted my perception of what I considered normal. And I was tired, tired, tired of such things. My original plan had been to analyze the literature and to conduct a scientific study of miscarriage. I had read all the experiments, had analyzed the results. I wanted to be done with it. As hindsight is apt to do, however, I don't think I had much of a choice.

When my final year of College rolled around, I struggled and fought with myself over which topic to devote a year to. My advisor seemed to sense my utter frustration. She told me to go to New York for the weekend and not to bring anything with me. So I did. As luck would have it, a hurricane had hit the city the day before and I got stuck in traffic while a tree was being cleared off the highway. So I sat. And I thought.

There was nowhere for me to go but inward. I started where I was and worked backwards. As I did, I realized that I was sitting in traffic because I had run away from the topic of miscarriage. I had run away from it because I just happened to get an internship and see what many women who have miscarriages experience but don't know about. I had gotten that internship because my interests in women's health had expanded from just pregnancy and birth. My interests had shifted because of my work at the OB/GYN. The decision to work in that environment came from my awareness of grief and loss and how it contrasted with my focus in birth. Birth had fascinated me because it was the end result of the mystery of pregnancy. And this curiosity stemmed all the way back to being twelve years old, sitting in a break room, and knowing that I did not know.

My mother was fascinated by this project in ways that I will probably never fully comprehend. In the middle of my research, she video chatted me to ask a question about her computer. In the lapses between me describing a button and mom trying to find it, I kept picking up books that I had read to tell her about it. She brought up the Dilation and Curettage that she had after her first miscarriage, and we started talking about how in my mind it was the most painless thing for the baby. This led to a conversation on the

6

difference between the perception of a baby and the expectation of a child. My mother remarked that she didn't think about it that often. Then she started crying. Then she told me just how often she did. What broke me down was not the ache that my mother carried around with her; it was the fact that such a hell had never been spoken of. Birthday after birthday, cousin after cousin; my mother was the aunt who stood behind the cake, took the family photos and never talked about what part of her was missing from all of it.

I asked her if it was the first time she had ever said anything about this. She responded by asking why she would in the first place. In the pause between the questions was my mother. In the pause after was the realization that I had not been her only child. I was, however, the only one she felt she was allowed to keep. I am the first person she has ever told her birth experience to. I am the first person she has ever told about the pain she gets when she thinks about the names that were destined, never used, and now marked forever. Where was her mother? Where were her sisters?

I was indignant about this for a few weeks until I realized: it was not that my mother didn't want to talk. She had never told anyone because no one had ever asked. From this point on, our relationship and my project completely shifted. We had broken some barrier, and with it came a new kind of dialogue. I think that it is very easy to think of our mothers, daughters and sisters as souls who exist within that role and that role only. When we talk about pregnancy loss, we have to acknowledge that these women have also lived roles that we will never understand. As it is human nature to prefer that which affects you, perhaps outsiders could approach involuntary pregnancy loss through the connections that they do have with it. We don't talk about that. But we should.

And I did. My official purpose of the project was to examine the experience of miscarriage by giving voice to the women within the involuntary pregnancy loss community. Through an ethnographic analysis I aimed to integrate literature, demographics, scientific findings, interviews, and a comparison between experiences in an effort to better understand the perceived silence and stigma around pregnancy loss before twenty weeks. Central to this, I wanted to identify:The cultural, sociopolitical, and historical factors that affect the perception of miscarriage in society as well as its influence on the woman's position within her community.

**The significance of the miscarriage experience when approached within the   context of the individual's entire reproductive history.

**A better understanding of the influence of community and support structures on a woman's perceived experience.

**The cultural norms and assumptions that differentiate the miscarriage community from the rest of society.

I also had several main questions:

**How does the female community (family, friends) that the woman is a part of play a role?

**How do age, parity, and family history play a role?

**How similar or different are individual women's experiences in comparison to the scientific literature?

I took advantage of many different resources to answer these questions. For a background and analysis of the miscarriage experience, I utilized scientific studies that have quantitatively and qualitatively approached the experience of pregnancy loss for women. To meet the authors of these papers as well as to learn about the newest published research, I attended the 2010 Perinatal Bereavement Conference. In addition to scientific studies, I also incorporated literature that helped to build a historical, cultural and political context within which to view my interview results.

In person and over the phone, I interviewed women who were at least eighteen years of age, had experienced an involuntary loss of a wanted pregnancy prior to twenty weeks gestation, and who had consented to be interviewed about their experience. The interviews consisted of two parts: a questionnaire to gauge general demographics, and an interview consisting of open-ended questions. The interviews were analyzed in terms of themes and similarity to the findings and experiences cited in the published literature. Within each theme, I also included a narrative from the women in order to create a platform for the telling of experiences.

Finding Stories

Once I had decided to interview women about their miscarriage experiences, I realized that I had to find them. After having this project approved by the Institutional Review Board at Hampshire College, I placed general ads on Craigslist and pregnancy loss forums. Although I received a few immediate responses, I did not obtain enough interviews to build a project around.

As I researched involuntary pregnancy loss resources around the area, I came across the local SHARE pregnancy loss support group. I contacted the facilitator about my project, but was not optimistic that I would even receive an email back. What I got was an immediately warm and enthusiastic response, an invitation into her home, a valuable discussion about what pregnancy loss is like in the area, and an offer to help recruit participants. Having never even met me, the facilitator had already started telling women she knew about my project. By the time I walked through her hazy blue kitchen and sat down on a rocking chair in the purple half-room to explain my background, several women had already expressed interest in telling me their stories. The next morning, I woke up to an inbox full of women offering to meet with me and tell me what had happened to them.

So, I met them. Twelve participants contacted me about my project. After giving informed consent, they were interviewed in person or over the phone between November 2010 and January 2011. Consent was obtained through a form that explained the procedures, possible risks and future visibility of the results. For phone interviews, the consent form was acknowledged, and vocal affirmation was recorded at the beginning of the conversation. We talked in coffee shops, in homes, and over the phone. Each interview changed my perspective just a little bit more. Not surprisingly, I ended up with more questions than I had started out with. Regardless, here is what I learned, who I learned it from, and how I learned it.

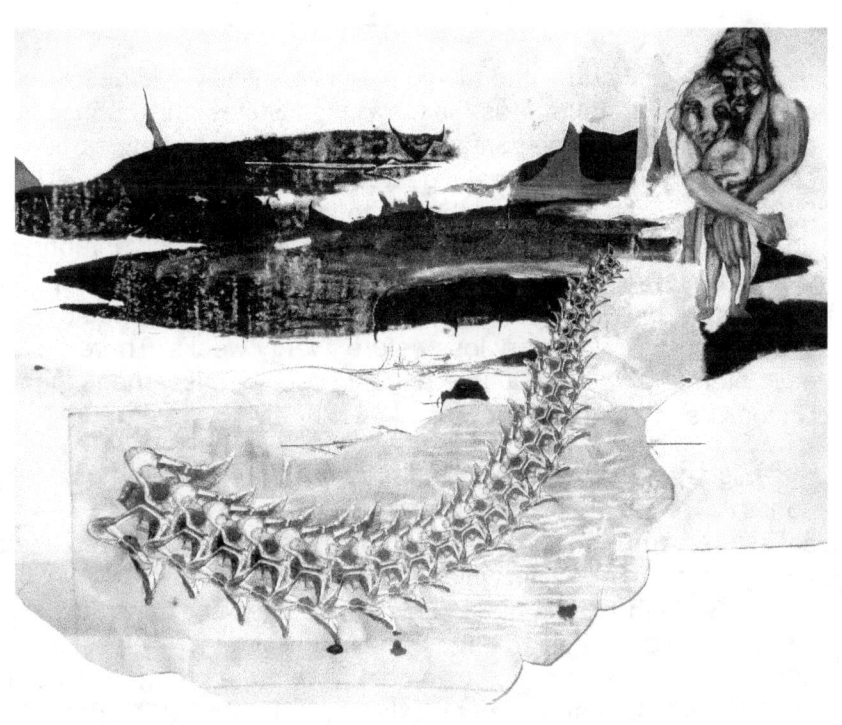

Part 1

Background

The Questionnaire

How exactly does the medical and scientific world describe involuntary pregnancy loss? In the United States, miscarriage is clinically defined as a spontaneous pregnancy loss between conception and twenty weeks gestational age (Swanson et al., 2007). Research has found that 15 to 20 percent of pregnancies end in miscarriage, but it may actually be 30 percent if unreported cases are included (Farquharson et al., 2005). This would mean that statistically, one in four women who become pregnant would experience an involuntary loss before twenty weeks. There are an estimated 600,000 to 800,000 annual cases of miscarriage in the United States annually (Bowles et al., 2000).

Miscarriage can be further defined as either a chromosomally abnormal or a chromosomally normal loss. Abnormal loss constitutes around half of all pregnancy losses and involves a fatal configuration of genetics which makes the fetus unviable (Weck et al., 2008). In this case, outside factors such as social health disparities are unlikely to have a role in the pregnancy loss. In normal loss there are no known defects and the pregnancy loss is more likely to be influenced by external factors. Even though involuntary pregnancy loss is defined as one of these two terms, the exact cause of the loss is often unknown (Neugebauer et al., 1996).

At the beginning of my research, these definitions seemed comprehensive and informative. As I continued to read articles and talk to women, however, inconsistencies and contradictions began to spring up. In her book, Motherhood Lost, Linda Layne (2003) found that:

> Many of these social scientific studies were quantitative and used various instruments to measure grief, depression and social support. And often they were 'action-oriented' toward care giving goals. On the whole, these studies focused on the individual and while several attempted to correlate social differences (level of education, marital status, etc.) with reactions to a loss, they have not analyzed pregnancy loss from a cultural point of view (22-23).

With this in mind, I expanded my research to include books, memoirs, and general guides, set the gestational limit for my interviews at twenty-four weeks and used the word "miscarriage" in

11

my advertisements. However, an email from the facilitator of the SHARE group about my language and parameters shed light on the disconnect between what is told and what is lived:

> As terminology matters a great deal to these women, I would suggest that either you change the parameters of your sample (to twenty weeks and before) or add "or stillbirth" after the word miscarriage on your document. Sorry to be picky, but I just happen to know a lot of women who, having delivered and held their very tiny babies, find it very offensive when their baby is called a miscarriage. In fact, I've come across many women who lose pregnancies at eighteen or nineteen weeks who personally don't refer to them as miscarriages at all.

The fact that no scientific paper or support book had alerted me to the fact that some women are offended by the term "miscarriage" points to a significant disconnect between the community providing support and the community receiving it. After several frustrating days of trying to figure out how to either work around the term or to use it, I decided that I would do both. The term "miscarriage" is used in this project, specifically when referring to literature and interviews with women who were comfortable with using it. Out of respect for those who are hurt by this word I also integrated the term "involuntary pregnancy loss" whenever it was appropriate.

For the first part of my interviews, I aimed to discover how the demographics in miscarriage research results compared to demographics in real life. To gain a theoretical and analytical sense of my sample, I asked the women to self-identify their age, race, gender, occupation, highest education level, and relationship status. On the scientific side of things, asking the women to state these factors rather than assuming them was a way to legitimize my results. For example, race and gender are social constructs and my analysis would be considered assumption if I had listed the women as Caucasian and female without first asking them to self identify. I also wanted to see how life factors (such as age and occupation) affected later answers about reproductive history and support. After getting my results, I compared them to the current literature on miscarriage.

<u>Demographics</u>

**How old are you currently?

The women I interviewed ranged from twenty-seven to fifty-three years old. I asked the women for their current age for several reasons. Advanced maternal age (over thirty-five) has been identified as a possible factor for the increased risk of miscarriage, and I was interested in possible correlations (La Rochebrochard and Thonneau, 2002). Although the mean age in my project was over thirty-five, most of the women had experienced their first miscarriage before reaching this cutoff. Of the five women I interviewed who were currently older than 35, two experienced their losses before reaching this age. In total, nine of the women interviewed experienced a loss before the age of thirty-five, which brings me to the general conclusion that advanced maternal age was most likely not a significant factor in my sample.

I was also interested in what age group would be most comfortable talking about their experiences. As per the Institutional Review Board, I did not specifically seek out women to interview. Rather, my information was displayed and distributed in a public and semi-public manner, and all of the women initiated contact. This allowed me to not direct my project at any one age group. I also refrained from advertising on college campuses in the area so as not to restrict my interviews to younger women. However, the age range in the SHARE group may influence the age of the women interviewed, as all of the women I talked to in the group were married and post college. My exclusion of unwanted pregnancies may also be a factor in the minimum age I encountered, as this rate is higher for younger women (Ventura et al., 2008).

**What race and gender do you identify with?

All twelve women identified themselves as white females. As I will show, race plays a significant role in miscarriage, but women of color are not well represented in the research about it. In fact, Van (2001) found that "There are no published studies about the healing strategies after pregnancy or infant loss for any ethnic/racial category of women" (231). The majority of studies that I read identified the women in their samples as Caucasian. For example, the sample group for *Affirming Motherhood: Lessons from Mothers'* *Narratives of Perinatal Hospice* consisted of fifteen couples, thirteen of which identified as Caucasian (Lanthrop, 2009). An article by Côte-Arsenault et al. (2004) had a sample group consisting of 90 percent white women with the remaining 10 percent identifying as Asian or Pacific Islander. This is definitely not an accurate representation of the general population: according to the 2010 United States Census, 72.4 percent of the American population identifies as white. This would mean that for any current research which addresses the general population, using sample groups that are 90-100 percent white leaves out 27.6 percent of the population (U.S Census Bureau, 2010).

When members of the pregnancy loss community do come together to discuss research and information, the topic of demographics and access within the sample groups is rarely brought up. When it is, discussions are more opinion than evidence based. For example, when the subject came up during Lanthrop's talk at the International Conference on Perinatal and Infant Death it was noted that the sample group was mostly Christian, but not that it was also mostly white. There was no discussion about the resources (time, income, support) needed to participate in a hospice program, or the lack of access that could have limited other families from choosing this path for the pregnancy (Lanthrop, 2009).

Part of this lack in awareness may stem from the makeup of the researchers themselves. For example, all of the facilitators of the Côte-Arsenault et al. (2004) study were white. At the 2010 International Perinatal Bereavement Conference in Alexandria VA, most of the group appeared to be white, and there were no workshops that specifically looked at the role of race and access in miscarriage. This is in keeping with Reagan's (2003) analysis of the representations of pregnancy loss in the 20th century. She found that "the [pregnancy loss support] movement's social location may explain why it universalizes emotions and values regarding miscarriage. Middle-class white women believe that they are the norm" (373).

**What is your occupation and highest education level?

Of the twelve women I interviewed, three women self-identified themselves as "stay at home moms", two women told me that they are currently looking for work, three women are editors, one woman is a social worker, one woman is a general district manager and dietician, and one woman is currently in school to become a Physician's Assistant. The highest education level ranged from some college education to a PhD. Two women had some college education, five women had a bachelor's degree, two women had obtained a masters degree, one woman had obtained a PhD, and two women were currently continuing their education after receiving their bachelors.

I asked for occupation and education level to analyze the overall social class of the women I talked to. Although I did not ask for specific income information, I took the level of education and current career or field as significant predictors of economic status. It costs money and time to pursue higher education, and all of the women I interviewed had at least some college experience.

This signified to me that the socioeconomic status of my sample might not reflect the general demographics of women who experience miscarriages. Instead, my results are similar to the samples used in the scientific literature. For example, in the article *"Support groups helping women through pregnancy after loss"* by Côte-Arsenault et al. (2004), the average annual income for the sample group was $60,000 to $79,000. This is a much higher average than $35,549, the 2009 ACS median annual earnings for women nationally (Getz, 2009). The sample also had an average of 16.5 years of education, with a minimum of 12 years (Côte-Arsenault et al., 2004). In contrast, the average level of education for an American in the twenty-five to thirty-nine year old age group (the mean age in the study was thirty-five) is 12.9 years (Kirsch, 2002).

Thoughts on Demographics

My sample did not significantly waiver from what the literature has reported in terms of race, class and relationship status. There are pros and cons to this. Having a similar demographic makeup as many of the studies I read allows me to compare the results within the context of a sample that is white, middle class, and in monogamous heterosexual relationships. The problem is that this is the only context I do have. What is ironic about the makeup of the samples in most of the studies is that the women used may have lower chances of experiencing a miscarriage because of their demographics. In fact, lower socioeconomic status, lower education level, identifying with a minority race and ethnicity, and chronic stress stemming from life events are all possible factors in causing a disproportionate level of involuntary pregnancy loss in the population (Neugebauer et al., 1996).

Lower socioeconomic status has been implicated as a significant factor of health disparities and perinatal loss (Price, 2006). For example, "*Prevalence and Correlation of Pregnancy Loss History In a National Sample of Children and Families*" used data from the Early Childhood Longitudinal Study, Birth Cohort (ECLS-B), to measure the frequency and correlation of pregnancy loss in women (who are currently parents) with racial and socioeconomic disparities. One quarter of the women in the database had experienced pregnancy loss (16.65 percent singular loss, 8.42 percent multiple losses). When these percentages were applied to demographics, socioeconomic status, race-ethnicity, and education levels were significantly correlated with increased rates of multiple involuntary pregnancy loss (Price, 2006).

Additionally, education levels are a significant factor in health outcomes and disparities (Freudenberg and Ruglis, 2007). Articles examining this relationship in the context of perinatal loss have found similar correlations. Parazzini et al. (1997) conducted a study to find evidence for risk factors of pregnancy loss during the first trimester and found a significant correlation between lower levels of education and higher levels of involuntary pregnancy loss.

Race and ethnicity have been shown to significantly influence pregnancy outcomes such as infant mortality and low birth weight (Collins and David, 2009). Its effect is also evident in the national perinatal loss rates. In addition to several other factors, Price (2006) found that there was a significant correlation between Black, non-Hispanic women and higher rates of involuntary pregnancy loss.

Studies, such as "*Association of Stressful Life Events With Chromosomally Normal Spontaneous Abortion*" by Neugebauer et al. (1996) have found a correlation between chronic stress and

16

higher rates of pregnancy loss. In addition to suggesting a difference in socioeconomic demographics between rates of chromosomally abnormal and chromosomally normal losses, women who had experienced a chromosomally normal pregnancy loss were more likely to be of a lower socioeconomic status, belong to a minority group, and be less educated.

If the only visible story within the involuntary pregnancy loss community is that of the white middle class woman, all experiences will be assumed to exist within that framework. To claim general knowledge from individual experience perpetuates the idea that " a woman's physical and emotional experiences provide her accurate knowledge about other women…" (Reagan, 2003:373). In keeping with this concept, I asked the women to describe the influences that set the context for their individual experiences through questions about location, religion, and family makeup.

Structures

**Do you have any religious affiliations? If so, what kind?

One woman identified herself as Jewish and three women identified themselves as Catholic. Three women identified themselves with the Church of Latter Day Saints, and five women had no current religious affiliations. Nine of the women currently hold the same affiliations they were raised with and three women currently hold different affiliations.

I asked questions about religion for several reasons. I was interested in the role that religion played in terms of support systems. Secondly, for women who did have strong religious affiliations, I was interested as to whether their loss would increase their belief and level of activity in their religion, or if it would cause anger and distance from the institution. Finally, I was interested in how different religions had different effects on the women who experienced losses. Within this, my main focus was on Catholicism and the Church of Latter Day Saints. Although women identified as religious, the detailed impact of their belief systems did not come up during the interviews. When asked about the role of their religious communities there was no major or consistent emphasis towards increased support or distance.

17

**What is your current state of residence? Where were you raised?

Seven women currently reside in Massachusetts. Four women currently reside in Utah. One woman currently resides in Rhode Island and Barcelona, Spain. Seven of the women currently reside in the state that they were raised in. Five of the women reside in a different area from where they were raised. My goal in asking this question was to gauge the significance of location and familiarity in the miscarriage experience. For the women who still reside in the state where they grew up, there tended to be a stronger sense of family support and contact. In contrast, the women who lived farther away from their hometown seemed to have more difficulties in gaining support.

**Do you have any siblings? If so, how many brothers and sisters do you have?

The number of siblings (including half-siblings) the women reported ranged from one to sixteen. Nine of the women had at least one sister. I asked women about their family size in an effort to gauge possible levels of support. I also asked how many sisters they had and specifically looked at the female community because miscarriage physically affects biologically female persons. These factors could influence how many people there are to talk to and how or if the family culture includes female community. A greater number of female siblings did not always seem to positively affect the experience. Rather, it was the amount and type of contact with these family members that made the difference.

Thoughts on Structure

In addition to understanding which support structures are in place for the women I interviewed, I wanted to gain an awareness of why these structures are important and how they can be strengthened. For example, information is beneficial if it prepares families for the possible reactions of their social networks. DeMontigny et al. (1999) argues that explaining to the woman and her family about the possible ways that their social network might react (such as not talking about the situation) and clarifying possible reasons for these responses (such as fear of upsetting the woman) may alleviate social conflicts.

From my research, I identified how these strategies statistically improve the current structures in the women's lives (Abboud et al., 2005, DeMontigny et al., 1999, Nikčević, 2003). Throughout my interviews, I used these findings as guidelines to gauge whether or not the women had a strong support system. In the literature, positive experiences resulted from allowing the family to talk about their experience and openly discuss their emotions and how the miscarriage has affected them, open dialogue with extended social networks about the acknowledgement of grief, defining emotions in clear language for dialogues, allowing partners to discuss their loss, suggesting rituals and ways in which the family can actively grieve if they choose to, and offering resources for long term support (DeMontigny et al., 1999). When I found evidence of these strategies in my results, they were consistently correlated with more positive experiences and increased healing.

In addition to demographics and support structure, reproductive history and outcomes played a major role in shaping the experiences of the women I talked to. To gain more of an understanding about which aspects of reproduction were the most significant, I inquired about the number of pregnancies experienced, when they occurred, what their outcomes were, how they differed from family history, the types of treatments they experienced, and reasons for their losses.

Reproductive History

**How many pregnancies have you experienced? What are the dates and outcomes of all previous pregnancies?

The number of known (self-identified) pregnancies experienced ranged from one to eleven. In total, there were thirty-four involuntary pregnancy losses in my interviews. Twenty-nine of these took place in the first trimester. Of the four that took place in the second trimester, three occurred after 19.0 weeks.

19

The number of losses per woman ranged from one to eleven. Four of the women experienced a single loss, three of the women experienced two losses and six women experienced three or more (defined as recurrent) losses. The gestational age at time of loss ranged from five to almost twenty weeks. Some self-reported losses were not medically confirmed and the gestational age is unknown. Eight of the women only experienced losses in the first trimester, two women only experienced losses in the second trimester and two women experienced losses in both trimesters.

Do you have any living biological children? If so, how many?

Three women do not currently have any living biological children. Three women have one living biological child, and four of the women have two or more living biological children. Additionally, two of the women were pregnant (one had no children, one had children) at the time of interview. I asked the women how many living children they currently had in an effort to gauge whether the loss was the only pregnancy experience the women had, or if they had also experienced successful live births. The amount of losses compared to other pregnancies, whether or not other pregnancies resulted in a successful live birth, and the order in which these pregnancies were experienced all seemed to play a significant role in how each miscarriage was experienced. This includes both the immediate reaction to the loss as well as the current state of awareness about its significance in their lives.

**Is there a history of pregnancy loss in your family? If so, what is the family member's relationship to you, and how many losses did they experience?

Out of the twelve women, five had no known history of pregnancy loss in their family. Five of the women's mothers had experienced at least one involuntary loss. Two women had grandmothers who had experienced a loss, and two had sisters who had experienced several losses. My goal in asking this question was to gauge whether or not the women had a family member that was also a part of the miscarriage community.

**What course of treatment did you take?

The delivery/induction methods used were labor induction, Dilation and Curettage (D and C), chemical induction (medication, also known as "medical treatment") and no medical treatment. Which method a woman ended up with was a result of the physical situation and their personal choice. In terms of physical factors, methods were chosen based on:

--The gestational age of their pregnancy

--How complete the miscarriage was considered

--The length of time the miscarriage was experienced

--How much blood had been lost

--Provider suggestion

In terms of personal choice, methods were chosen based on:

--Trust of the medical provider's advice

--Past history with involuntary loss

--Negative past experiences with certain methods,

--Personal beliefs about the body

--Personal need to be physically being aware of the process

The fact that the type of treatment did not seem to significantly affect the emotional state of the women I talked to is similar to results in the literature. A study by Nielsen at al. (1996) randomly assigned 86 women undergoing treatment for a miscarriage before thirteen weeks to either undergo a Dilation and Curettage (D and C) or more conservative treatment (no surgical or medical intervention). Fourteen days after the miscarriage, the researchers found no significant difference between the groups in terms of "psychological reactions" (1767).

**Do you know if your loss was a result of a genetic defect?

The involuntary pregnancy losses in this project can be divided into three categories: genetic and chromosomal abnormalities, physical occurrences, and unknown:

--Two women experienced losses as a result of known chromosomal and genetic abnormalities. This included Trisomy 13, a blighted ovum, and a "chromosomal defect".

--Losses because of physical occurrences were premature rupture of membranes (pre prom) and pre-term labor (cause unsure). Each woman experienced an individual loss after 19 weeks gestational age.

--Eight women did not know if their loss was the result of a genetic abnormality. The loss fell under the category of unknown. This encompasses losses that were tested and had inconclusive results, losses that women chose not to test, and losses that women were not able to test because of finances or the situation.

Thoughts on Reproductive History

One of the most striking aspects of this project was the incredible difference the existence of another living biological child has on the miscarriage experience. Why did this have such an impact? The answer lies in the significance of reproduction within the context of being a woman and a member of society. Children are a sign of accomplishment and a powerful way to showcase one's genes, one's reproductive capabilities, and one's right to identify as a woman.

Historically, a woman's prime responsibility was to "lead a life that protected her ovaries and uterus" (Weitz, 2003: 274). Reproduction was both a fulfillment of responsibility as well as the only opportunity for a woman to exert power within her sphere. Additionally, influences such as religion shaped the options for women. For example, Sumrall and Vecchione, (1992) found that "Catholicism provides girls with only one narrow concept of womanhood: The 'virgin'-who is emblematic of modesty, purity, passivity, submission-the silent one who obeys God and yet is the mother of God, the one who has value not by virtue of her selfhood but by virtue of her function" (4).

A woman therefore had two options: she could choose to follow what had been declared her divine responsibility; or she could remain without children and in sin. There were consequences for failing to carry a pregnancy to term. For some communities, "miscarriage was seen as evidence of guilt"; in these cases a woman was shunned, divorced or even burned alive after losing a pregnancy (Reinharz, 1988:85). In the community's eyes, she had failed in her responsibility, lost the chance to gain control and invalidated her position as a true woman. Such reactions also served as an impetus to hide one's involuntary pregnancy loss from the public.

Although womanhood and motherhood have been correlated historically, one must also address whether or not the current drive to have children is a purely physical instinct or a completely constructed expectation of culture. I would argue that both play a role. Although the female body is biologically designed for pregnancy, the historical correlations and responsibilities of woman as mother give strong evidence to the influence that cultural expectation also has on the need for children.

In the past forty years, the childfree movement has attempted to break the bond between the definition of motherhood and womanhood. Their goal was to change the cultural mindset to view motherhood as a choice rather than an inevitable conclusion. The movement argued that expectations of reproduction are "an unconscious response to pressures that still predominantly define a woman's role and being in terms of motherhood" (Alizade, 2006:2). Their efforts influenced the gradual shift of cultural expectations, and it became acceptable for women to choose whether or not to have children. Or so it seemed. The childfree movement and our assumptions that motherhood is an individual autonomous choice forgot that "The basic paradigms of psychism do not change with the changing of customs, and one or two generations are certainly not sufficient to transform the foundations of our theory" (Alizade, 2006:16).

At first glance, the stories of the women I talked to appear to involve a decision to reproduce that was personal and independent of outside factors. However, if every woman is making the same choice, it raises the question of whether it is hers to make. Rather, it is an option and an acknowledgement that reproduction is an integral aspect of the female identity. If the actions of the individual are seen as a reflection on society as a whole, what can be construed as an individual desire to have children may in reality be a utilitarian expectation to keep one's community and culture intact.

Society may no longer have such strict requirements about the role of motherhood, but the expectation that one is capable of reproducing still dominates. For example, the childfree movement argues that the cultural approval of having children confines women to an ideal that imposes the role of motherhood and continues the dominance of patriarchy (Rich, 1976). However, in basing an argument on the assumption that birth always follows pregnancy, one actually continues the idea that womanhood is contingent upon motherhood. For example, "…the woman who does not have children through choice can at least buoy her femaleness by saying ' I could have a child if I wanted one" (Chase and Rogers, 2001:212). There is a difference between women who don't want to and women who can't, and no one knows that better than the women I met.

The Women

In addition to the analysis, I think that it is important that each woman is given a space to tell their own story within the context of their specific circumstances. What follows is my personal interpretation of the situations where the interviews took place as well as my best attempt to describe the women's stories as they were told to me.

Lisa

Lisa was one of the women who got my name from the SHARE facilitator and emailed me to be interviewed. We met on a very not sunny afternoon and conducted the interview in one of the video carrels at Hampshire College. As this was my first interview I was completely terrified. From the looks of it, so was Lisa. Her experience was still fresh, and telling it was very emotional. Here is what happened:

Lisa started her first pregnancy in April of 2008, which resulted in a loss at 19 weeks. About eight weeks into the pregnancy, she started having bleeding:

> *...They found a blood clot in my uterus. But they weren't really that concerned about it so they just kind of monitored it. I was on bed rest...[until]...fourteen weeks...[when] they took me off bed rest and I had no restrictions. The blood clot, they said it was so small that I wouldn't even know I had it. They felt pretty confident that I would be okay.* **Lisa**

A week after her restrictions were lifted, Lisa and her family went on a trip to Puerto Rico. At around 17 weeks and three days into the vacation, her water broke:

> *So I headed to the hospital in San Juan and...the first thing that they wanted me to do was just abort the baby. Even though the baby's vitals and everything were fine, just my water broke. I refused to do that so I was put on bed rest...they thought I was just going to go into spontaneous labor, I guess that's common for when your water breaks. About four or five days later...it seemed as though my water was trying to accumulate again. So they were pretty*

*surprised and elated for that and my cervix was tight and closed and it [the fluid] was trying to re-accumulate so they thought everything would be okay...but the next day it seemed as though there was another tear or something happened and the water stopped accumulating so there was really no fluid there... **Lisa***

Lisa negotiated with her doctor and insurance company back home in Massachusetts, and the decision was made to Life-Flight her back home. She was hospitalized and placed on bed rest until 19 weeks, when:

*...They finally convinced me that I had to induce labor because if the baby were to be born they didn't think she would be able to survive...so at 19 weeks they induced labor and she was born and she died in childbirth... **Lisa***

She went on to have a very early loss in In January or February of 2009, and a full term birth on April 28th, 2010. From the looks of the picture she showed me on her phone, her daughter is quite a happy child.

Jennifer

Jennifer was my second interview. She had contacted me through a Craigslist ad I had placed. We met in a bright and unfortunately noisy café one morning in town. I was interested to know why she had decided to be interviewed. She told me that she was a supporter of student research and was happy to help out whenever she could. I am not sure if it was the fact that we were in such a public place, but many of Jennifer's answers were short and to the point. Here is what she told me:

Jennifer started her first pregnancy in 1994, which resulted in a loss at 8 weeks. When I asked her to tell me about her experience with pregnancy loss she told me that she had really been looking forward to this pregnancy:

...We got married in January. [We had been married] just one year in that time [that I got pregnant]. So I was really excited about the pregnancy...at eight weeks [I] started bleeding and spotting and didn't know why. So I went to the

midwife…[she] said it was definitely a miscarriage so I had to go home and wait for it to pass…I didn't want to hear that it was a definite miscarriage; I was in denial about that. So I resented them telling me that it was. **Jennifer**

Jennifer went on to have a full term birth in 1995. She thinks about the pregnancy all of the time, but does not really talk about it much. And that is all I know.

Cindy

Cindy was my third interview. She had also contacted me on Craigslist, and we had set up a time to meet in a café that I was not familiar with. After talking to Jennifer, I was worried that meeting in a public place would result in Cindy not being able to open up about what happened. I got there early, ordered coffee, and anticipated the story ahead. The act of waiting for someone you have never seen yet knowing exactly who they are when they walk in is a strange feeling, but it definitely happened every time I had to meet a woman to interview. Then again, it cannot be hard to miss the college student sitting alone with a nervous look and an informed consent sheet.

My interview with Cindy was something I did not expect. After Lisa's story I assumed talking to women would always be fraught with sadness. After Jennifer I was worried that women were not going to open up to me if they were interviewed in a public place. Cindy laughed throughout what seemed the entire interview. She possessed an air of "what happens happens." I remember driving home afterwards and feeling not quite excited, but very full of hope and possible confidence that every interview was going to completely change how I perceived the world. Cindy told me the story of her miscarriage within the context of her life. When she was young, she travelled the country with a mattress in the back of her truck. She was a reformed lapsed Catholic. She had babies, and she lost some too. Here is what happened:

Cindy had her first pregnancy, which resulted in a full term birth, in 1981. Her next pregnancy resulted in a miscarriage at ten weeks on St. Patrick's Day of 1995. She told me, "*That was a girl.*" When I asked her about her experience with this loss, she responded:

...The question was always...they didn't know if the baby died because I got sick or if I got sick because the baby died... I came home from work that day [because] I [had] started feeling lousy at work. I had a doctor's appointment the next morning so I didn't bother doing anything. I was cramping up, [I had a] fever. I just...we weren't really sure what was going on but...we weren't too worried about it...when we got into the hospital...I remember having the ultrasound. And the ultrasound tech...I know there's something wrong because I can tell by the look on her face...all of a sudden she stopped talking. And she was acting really weird and then she left the room. I was like 'okay so now I have to wait for the doctor to decide to come in'. It took a really long time, you know...and then they came in and they told me and they said you got to have a D and C...you know, I don't ask personal questions usually, so I didn't know anything about it. So that was an experience in itself (laughs)...it was just a really weird experience. **Cindy**

Cindy went on to have full term live births in April of 1998 and November of 1999. She told me that after the second pregnancy, they had her "down for two more miscarriages", which were most likely around seven weeks.

Jenn

Jenn was my fourth interview. I had placed an ad on a pregnancy loss website to see if anyone would be interested. No one responded for the first few days, so I was surprised to get an email two weeks later. Jenn lived in Utah, so she was my first phone interview. From 2003 until 2010, she had seven pregnancies and three full term births. Here is what happened:

Jenn's first pregnancy resulted in a full term birth on November 11th, 2003. Her next pregnancy ended in a loss at eight weeks in April of 2005. Her third pregnancy ended in a loss at six weeks in October of 2005. Her fourth pregnancy resulted in a full term birth on July 2nd, 2008. Her fifth pregnancy resulted in a loss at fifteen weeks that was discovered at 19 weeks. She then had a full term pregnancy that resulted in a birth on August 29th, 2009. This was followed by a pregnancy that ended in loss in October of 2009 at seven weeks. When I asked her to describe her general experience with pregnancy loss, she responded:

> ...Disheartening, I guess...the hardest one was the last one. I think [it] was probably the most traumatic...just because it was so many, and having children around...I had two boys already so I really wanted a girl. After I delivered the doctor said he was 99 percent sure it was a girl. From what he could tell so...that was really hard. It was also a really stressful time...I was working a lot and I was with my other kids already so it was a pretty...hard impact. The two miscarriages that I had in a row were hard because even after, it was two in a row and after that it took me eight months to get pregnant again. *Jenn*

Because she had mentioned that the later loss was the most traumatic, I asked her to tell me more about the experience. She responded:

> That was the one that took me by surprise because that was later. And I had my doctor's appointment at fourteen weeks and heard the heartbeat, and then...my next appointment, which was when we were supposed to find out [whether] we were having [a boy or girl], it was found out. *Jenn*

Susan

Susan was my fifth interview. She had contacted me through Carol and we agreed to meet at a Starbucks. This time, I was the one who recognized her. She was sitting at a large table holding a coffee cup in both hands and looking around for someone. Our interview was hampered by how public the area was, but Susan seemed very happy to open up as much as she could about her story. Up until this point, all of the women I had talked to had at least one living child. Susan did not. The interview left me confused at how things just don't always work out. I felt like a small child who had just been told her first bedtime story without a happy ending. The other experiences had been sad, but they had also worked out in the end. Here is what happened:

Susan's first pregnancy resulted in a loss at ten weeks in September of 2008. For four years until that point, she and her husband had been trying in vitro fertilization:

...We went through fertility treatment, we went through IUI and then IVF...And at that point I had given up hope, I was like 'whatever'. But the doctors said you [should] have a blood test anyway. And it came out positive. And so we checked and there was a heartbeat...then about a month later I was camping. I felt a little weird so I...I had tons of blood and...I was really upset...Tuesday morning I went into the ultrasound. I was still pregnant and the heartbeat was still there...they couldn't give me an explanation for what happened. So yeah...a few days later I started bleeding and at that point they told me that there was no heartbeat anymore. Susan

Susan told me that her insurance would no longer cover fertility treatments. That was it. As Susan puts it, "it would be nice to have a biological child, but you know it's not going to happen..." She is now in the process of adopting. Unlike the other women I talked to, her narrative is much more of a moment past than of one that continues.

Jenni

Jenni was my sixth interview. She had contacted me through Carol, and we had agreed that I would come to her house. I was a little nervous, but was very warmly welcomed. Jenni had been baking, and the color, lighting, and smell of her kitchen and living room was a great contrast from the snow and December outside. Perhaps it was the fact that we were in her home, but Jenni really seemed to open up in telling her story. I remember thinking during the interview about how I wished all of my interactions could take place in this type of setting. Here is what happened:

Jenni's first pregnancy was in 1998 and resulted in a termination. Her second pregnancy began in October 2008. It resulted in a loss in February 2009 just before twenty weeks:

I'm pretty newly married. So I actually [got] pregnant on my honeymoon and it wasn't... particularly planned but it also wasn't particularly avoided...We had talked about it but not thoroughly...So I didn't really do any kind of prenatal care or prenatal planning. It was like 'we were in love, we were getting married, throw caution to the wind'. And I ended up getting pregnant. I bled for most of the pregnancy because

30

of the [cervical] polyp so I didn't have…I never really had the experience of like. 'I'm pregnant and I'm sure that there's going to be a baby at the end of this' because…there was never a point where my body felt like it had really stabilized with the pregnancy…It wasn't induced. I actually went into preterm labor and had a baby pretty quickly. There wasn't actually the option of stopping labor. So the baby, the baby died during the laboring process…the baby was so early that she couldn't have been considered a micro preemie because it wasn't even twenty weeks yet. But what I physically went through is a very fast labor and delivery as opposed to a bleeding kind of situation. **Jenni**

Jenni's interview was similar to Susan's in that she had not yet experienced a successful live birth. However, unlike Susan, Jenni is still trying to have a biological child.

Amy

Amy was my seventh interview. At this point in my project, I had gone to stay in New York City for a few weeks. On my way down, a friend called and told me that her mother would like to be interviewed. I had already done a phone interview, so I was a little less nervous this time. However, Amy was the first woman I had talked to that I had a connection to other than through her pregnancy loss. Here is what happened:

Amy's first pregnancy ended in a miscarriage at 8 weeks in 1988:

The first one had been [on] Christmas day…it was just very sudden…it was just…so long ago. It was traumatic but they were just so kind in the hospital and so nice and so understanding and…they tried to make me as comfortable as possible. And I felt like I was…young; I was twenty-eight years old and I really felt like 'okay I can cope with this'. It didn't seem like it was that terrible. It was early on enough in the pregnancy that it wasn't really devastating emotionally. We were really, really sad but we weren't feeling like 'oh God this is just a bad omen of things to come'. **Amy**

Amy's second pregnancy resulted in a loss on May 5th, 1989. This loss had much more of an impact on her:

But then the second one, I was at work…and I started bleeding and I just…that one really upset me because I [had] felt like 'okay I'm right, I'm about to start my second trimester and that means smooth sailing from here on'…the general common knowledge is that…if you make it through the trimester you're pretty much going to be okay…I just remember lying on my back in my office at work. Just, just thinking, 'oh I hope this isn't happening, I hope this isn't happening, I can't believe this is happening'. And I called my doctor and we had an ultrasound done right away and it showed that the fetus was no longer alive. And then I had to go to her office and she did a D and C while I was awake. And I just remember feeling…that it was just awful and it was physically and emotionally really painful and just…really devastating-and it was on my mother's birthday too. **Amy**

Amy's third pregnancy was her "lucky one" and resulted in a live birth on June 3rd, 1990. Her fourth pregnancy ended in a miscarriage in 1992 at nine weeks. Her fifth and final pregnancy resulted in a live birth in 1994.

Lexi

Lexi was my eighth interview, though she was scheduled to be one of the first women to tell me her story. She had contacted me through Carol and we had set up a date, but changes in plans meant that I interviewed her when she was twenty-three weeks pregnant rather than seventeen. It also meant that instead of meeting face to face in a café in December, I sat in Brooklyn in January and interviewed her over the phone in Massachusetts. The fact that we conducted the interview while she was driving may have made the interview better. As she explained:

I sort of began just jotting down thoughts to talk through and I realized that sometimes that's kind of a waste of time because when you put your writer brain on you get very linear…then when you're actually stopping and thinking, I'm driving right now, which is good for non linear thinking. **Lexi**

Here is what happened:

Lexi's first pregnancy ended on Thanksgiving of 2009 at nine weeks.

My first pregnancy...began after having tried for several months...we were trying for about 8 months. And just as sort of a general background, my professional work has always been in parenting publishing. [I've] actually [been] a pregnancy editor for the past two years. And I have quite a bit of...textbook knowledge about pregnancy and labor and delivery and [have gone] through doula training. So it is kind of an area that I have had a life long interest in professionally. So getting pregnant was sort of troublesome at first. We were at first really thrilled when it happened. And when my pregnancy ended, I think everything just kind of got very...dull for a while. And I really kind of let the color drain from the world for a long time. I opted not to have a D and C. and I was physically fine pretty much immediately. I was taking some herbs to expel the fetus. I recovered physically very quickly. And I just [felt] a lot of...residual sadness and [I felt] pretty isolated I would say. **Lexi**

Her second pregnancy ended on Easter of 2010 at five weeks:

And so my second pregnancy was definitely something that we unfortunately didn't know about. I had been told to wait several months to begin trying again and my husband and I were actively not trying. And so I had a period that lasted [a] very, very long [time], three weeks. And my acupuncturist finally cornered me and said 'I want you to take a pregnancy test. It's really important that you do this.' I was pregnant and I was also miscarrying. So that was really confusing and disheartening, and [a] really sad time...I definitely was not in the headspace where I had known I was pregnant; [I] didn't know that I was miscarrying...[I had a] certain mistrust of what my body was doing. So that was a really difficult place, especially after I felt like I had been through some really transformative experiences in those months. I was tired from going through the first loss. **Lexi**

Lexi became pregnant for the third time in August of 2010. Lexi was the first woman I interviewed who was currently pregnant, and I think the point she was at in the nine-month period really had an impact on her story.

33

Malissa

Malissa was my ninth interview. I had originally planned to interview women in New York City and Amherst, Massachusetts in an effort to see if location made a difference. As hard as I tried, I did not get any responses for New York. I put out an open request for women on Facebook, and Jenn responded. She referred me to several women, and one of them was Malissa. Her story is similar to Susan's in how it forcefully reminded me that life is not tidy. Here is what happened:

Malissa's first pregnancy occurred ten years ago, and ended in a miscarriage at twelve weeks. Her second pregnancy took place six months later, was ectopic, and ended at twelve weeks. Her third pregnancy was *"very quick...I had barely missed my period and miscarried."* Perhaps it was because these experiences took place so long ago, but Malissa's story was quite confusing. When I asked her about her experience, she responded:

> *I was in a relationship and we had tried to have kids for a long time and we just, nothing had happened. And of course we found out that I had all sorts of fertility issues. We had been together eight years and...suddenly I had this horrific pain. And it turns out I was having a miscarriage...finally one night I decided that I was going to the emergency room. It wasn't even a whole emergency room. It was just a little instacare type thing. And just that I'm experiencing a lot of abdominal pain. And they said well is it due to pregnancy and I was like 'yeah right, no (laughs), like that's even going to happen'. And so first thing they had me do is take a pregnancy test and getting in the doctor was like 'You're pregnant'. And I was said...'I don't believe you'. He's like 'well...you're pregnant and there's nothing we can do here. We have to send you to an ER'. Malissa*

She then described the course of the next two weeks that resulted in her completing the miscarriage on her own. Her second experience was described as:

> *...Kind of the same thing. I was spotting and it...just wasn't normal and so I thought 'oh I'm going to take a pregnancy test'. I took it and it was positive. And then I immediately*

34

*called my doctor the next morning and told him 'I have a positive pregnancy test and I'm spotting'. And he said 'okay, get in here'. And so I went in and…we kind of, it was kind of the same exact thing where he… did my blood work and did the ultrasound to see what he could see. He was able to determine really quickly that it was tubal. Due to pain location…and [it was] the same thing where…he had me you know, test my HCG levels for a few days just to see what they were doing. And they just gradually went up and…and that's when he said I was at risk for [losing] the whole fallopian tube altogether if I didn't get that taken care of so. So…he said 'I can give you the shot', so we did and… that took care of that. **Malissa***

For her third pregnancy:

*I had just missed my period and I, I could tell something was wrong with this one. Something was different; it was just different. It felt different. The blood was different. There were chunks so the color was different, everything. And…so I asked him [the naturopath] to check it and he said yeah. That I was…having a miscarriage. **Malissa***

However, later on in the interview, Malissa apologized and told me that:

*I haven't thought about this in a really long time…I'm going to go back and change my story, just change my facts a little… so the week and a half period, that was the tubal pregnancy. **Malissa***

I ended the interview unsure of what exactly had happened. But then again, Malissa wasn't either.

Amber

Amber was my tenth interview. Like Malissa, she had also contacted me through Jenn and we scheduled a phone interview. As she was pregnant at the time of interview, I found a lot of similarities between Amber and Lexi. Here is what happened:

Amber's first pregnancy ended in February 2005 at seven weeks:

I was just doing the wait and see but then I started bleeding a lot. So they ended up having to do an emergency D and C...the two that I lost were really close together. It was kind of a surprise. We had told everyone, like with my first one, we told everyone I was pregnant as soon as I found out. And so that was kind of hard after. We had to go tell everybody that I wasn't pregnant anymore. And then, it was a little traumatic with the emergency room visit; with the emergency D and C with all the bleeding it was...it was kind of scary. **Amber**

Her second pregnancy ended at around six weeks in April of 2005:

It was a little harder because I didn't actually know I was pregnant until I had the miscarriage... when the second one happened just a couple months later, it was...I didn't really know what was happening at first. **Amber**

Her third pregnancy ended with a live birth in August of 2007. She is currently in her fourth pregnancy. At the time of the interview she was thirty-one weeks pregnant.

Shannon

Shannon was my eleventh interview. She got my name through Carol, but didn't contact me until I was close to the end of the interviews. I sent her the questions to look over, and she sent them back to me answered. As a result the interview was much more of a review of what she had said then of what she had to say. She had experienced several losses over the past few years, nine for sure and eleven possibly. In response to how her first pregnancy affected her, she responded:

I was a wreck. Technically my first loss was a termination. At 19 weeks Isabella measured only thirteen to fourteen weeks because of severe intra-uterine growth restriction. There was also a risk of neural tube defects among other issues seen in a level-2 ultrasound. **Shannon**

After her first loss, Shannon experienced a string of first trimester losses. As she describes it:

*It took several months to get pregnant again but even when it happened I couldn't really be happy. I was filled with dread and worry and wondered when the other shoe would drop. I went in for an ultrasound and there was no heartbeat. I was scheduled for a D and C later in the week but began bleeding the next day and passed everything…after my second pregnancy I had a series of "chemical pregnancies" over nearly two years. **Shannon***

Kirsten

Kirsten was my twelfth and last interview. She had been connected to me through Jenn, and we talked over the phone. Her story was a good one to end my interviews with. Interesting things happen when you do not see the person who is talking. These stories have been swirling in my head for months. For the women whom I met in person, their face is very connected to their experience. But for the women whose faces I could not see, the tone of their voice made a much larger impact. Kirsten spoke softly and gently, but what words she chose were used with conviction. Here is what happened:

Kirsten's first pregnancy resulted in a miscarriage at eleven weeks in November 2006:

*Well the first pregnancy loss was very, very difficult for me. It was also the first pregnancy. **Kirsten***

Kirsten's second pregnancy ended in a live birth in January of 2006. Her third pregnancy resulted in a miscarriage at thirteen weeks in April 2006:

*…[During] the second pregnancy loss…I just felt like [I wanted] the more natural approach. I don't know if it was because I had another baby already [and] I didn't really feel ready for another, but it wasn't as bad for me. I just kind of allowed the experience to happen…it wasn't so bad because I felt like I…experienced it all myself and watched the way my body handled it. It just seemed to be a better way for me to handle it. **Kirsten***

Kirsten's fourth and most recent pregnancy resulted in a live birth in February 2009.

Part 2

Narratives

By the end of my interviews I had collected twelve distinct, detailed and personal tales about involuntary pregnancy loss. The question was, how would I use their words to emphasize possible commonalities as well as the importance of individual experience? I broke my questions up into two forms: the first focused mainly on quantitative data, and these questions were usually finished within the first ten minutes. It was the second part of my interviews, the open ended questions, where I started to gain more of an understanding of involuntary pregnancy loss, the community around it, and what silence really means. After compiling the transcripts together, I read through all of them at once in order to connect a common narrative. From there, I broke the narrative up into themes with a discussion at the end of each section. This allowed me to create a space to let the women speak for themselves. And they did. Their words developed into Milestones, Power, Pain, Stigma, and Distance. My analysis of these narratives and themes is not meant to be a final conclusion about every involuntary pregnancy loss experience. Rather, it is my effort to bear witness to the factors that affected the women who shared their stories. It is my hope that the lessons learned from these themes will serve as a starting point to understanding and supporting women who experience an involuntary pregnancy loss.

<u>Milestones</u>

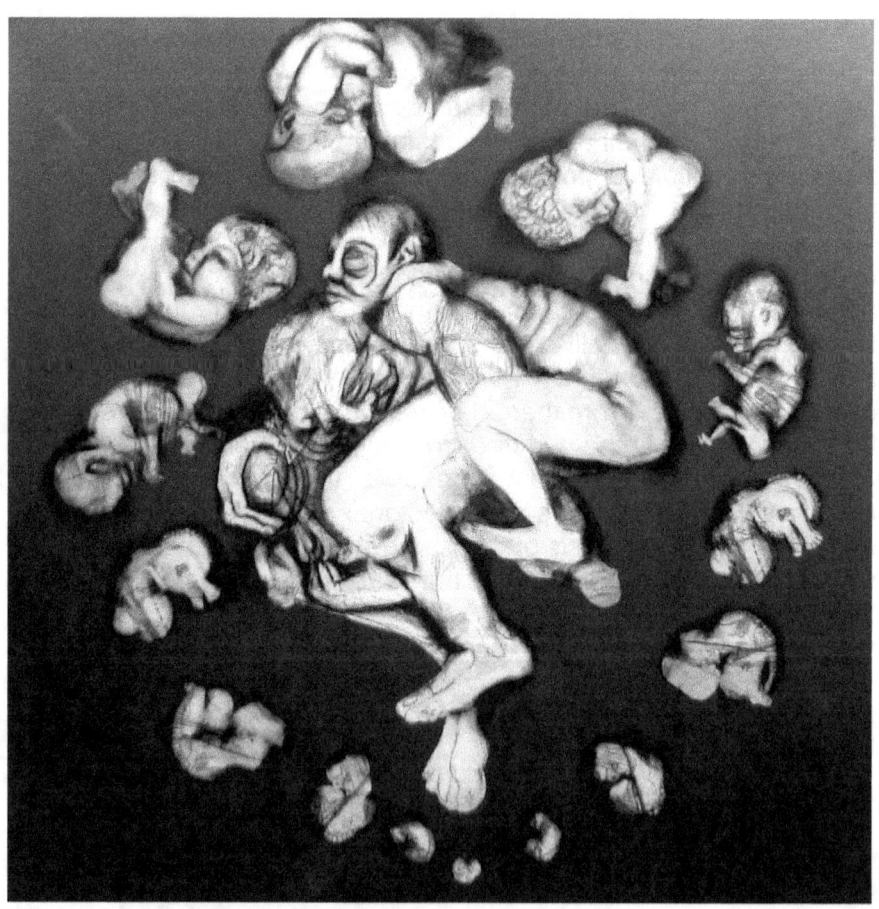

Pregnancy is a state of waiting. In order to conceptualize our proximity to its end result, we often describe gestation through the use of milestones and in terms of its progression. A specific moment can only be understood within the context of what came before and what will come after. Trimesters and weeks therefore play a very significant role in how we validate the pregnancy as a real state with a concrete result. They are fundamental to the validation of what is becoming, and in the case of miscarriage, what would have been.

Miscarriage itself is also a milestone. As is evident by the stories of the women who were interviewed, factors such as age, other pregnancies, dates, and life events shaped the type of experience and the mark it made on the woman's reproductive timeline. All of these aspects came up again and again in my interviews with women. I specifically found them in the difference in medical treatment for miscarriage and stillbirth, in the perception that everything will be fine after the first trimester, in the correlation between gestational age and how much the pregnancy counts, in the proximity of the date of loss with other significant dates, in the correlation between perceived significance of loss and the length of time since the event, and in the age of the woman. Although opinions differed at certain points there is no doubt that the timing of the miscarriage shapes the role of the experience in a woman's life.

A twenty-week wall: the significance of gestational age at time of loss

The medical community defines an involuntary loss after the twentieth week of pregnancy as a stillbirth (Kowaleski, 1997). As I saw in the labor and delivery ward at Mount Sinai, some hospitals keep a manual for such a situation. As per instruction, the "baby" is dressed and the parents are allowed to take time to say goodbye. A stillbirth is, for all intents, purposes, and ceremonies, a death. On the other hand, a loss before twenty weeks seems to be nothing more than a miscarriage. For the women I interviewed who experienced losses near to the twenty-week mark, this gestational limit makes all the difference. Especially for Lisa:

> *And a horrible thing is that I could have waited to induce labor; I could have waited another few days and it would have been twenty weeks. And then she would have had a birth certificate. But because I did it before then she was just, she was just a miscarriage. And it's like I can't look at that as a miscarriage because it wasn't in any sense of the word.*
> **Lisa**

Loss near the twenty-week mark is additionally difficult in the sense that it does not fit with the general idea of what a miscarriage is:

40

It's hard especially in my case where I had a preconceived notion that a miscarriage was, you know, you're eight weeks and all of a sudden you get your period. And I don't think it's fair...I can only say that because I lost at nineteen weeks but for someone who lost [at] twelve weeks and feels the same way that I felt...But I'm, that's what I picture of a miscarriage so it was really upsetting when I was termed a miscarriage... **Lisa**

As women told me their experiences with medical care I began to piece together how a loss before twenty weeks is treated. In contrast, Jenni's experience allowed me to see how loss after twenty weeks is approached:

We actually really, the one place we lucked out with our medical care was that we ...mostly because [my husband] lied, which was kind of awesome (laughs). When he called the hospital we told them that we were coming in and that we were twenty weeks pregnant. But we were actually a couple days shy. And so they let me into L[abor] and D[elivery] rather than the ER. Which I really feel is one of the most insane rules. That if you aren't twenty weeks pregnant you can't access L and D because really what is the different between twenty-four, or forty-eight, or seventy-two hours and the development of the child...You can be attended by ER staff or you can be attended by a midwife. It's crazy. **Jenni**

Jenni's experience also casts light on the incredible difference a few days make:

I went into L and D and there was an on call midwife who was fantastic with us...I delivered very quickly. Like within ten minutes of getting in the door. She [the midwife]...got the nurses in line in terms of this is a person having a baby and so we need to treat her like she's having a baby. And so, you know. They washed the baby and they dressed her and they wrapped her in a blanket and they gave her a little hat and they wheeled her in on a cart and they put her in my arms and it was like the whole ritual of 'you have had a baby' that we got to do with her...they took her hand and footprints. They made a little box with her things [and] they took her measurements. They wrote a condolence note and they gave her the information...the way we were treated was a lot as if we had had a stillbirth. **Jenni**

There are some differences on either side of the twenty-week wall. I had first made contact with Lexi when she was seventeen weeks pregnant, but we were unable to do the interview until she was twenty-three weeks. When we did talk I asked her how she thought the conversation would have been different if we had done the interview right away. She responded:

I have to say that at seventeen weeks...I hadn't felt the baby move yet and I was still beyond sick. Just sick, sick...sick. And so I would probably have been in super low spirits. Not especially optimistic about how things were turning out. I wish there was a way to turn off that limbic brain that [is] dangling all of these possibilities at you all the time. But especially in my first sixteen or seventeen weeks I wasn't able to do that. And now I can go two or three days without ever thinking 'oh, well it might not, you know, in theory were going to have the baby but it might now work out'. I can now shop for strollers. I can...think about baby names. I do normal quote unquote pregnancy things, which I... I don't think I was doing that at seventeen weeks. **Lexi**

The official terminology and timing of pregnancy loss varies and is erratic in both scientific literature and general information. For example, in a review of the medical articles on this topic, Wright (2010) found that the "Last Taboo" (miscarriage) was understudied, with inconsistencies in both terminology used and evidence. Phrases that are used interchangeably include miscarriage, spontaneous abortion, pregnancy loss, missed abortion, and perinatal loss. However, these phrases have very different definitions. To miscarry is defined in the Miriam-Webster dictionary as failure "to achieve the intended purpose" (Merriam-Webster 2010). In contrast, a spontaneous abortion is defined as " a natural loss of the products of conception" (Merriam-Webster 2010).

Facts such as the official gestational limit are also inconsistent in the biomedical community. This is especially evident when literature is compared by country. British researchers Rai and Regan (2006) define miscarriage as an involuntary pregnancy loss up to twenty-four weeks. However, American researchers Swanson et al. (2007) cite Ventura et al. (2000) in defining miscarriage as an involuntary pregnancy loss up to twenty weeks. Viability is generally accepted as the divide between a miscarriage and a stillbirth. Seri and Evans (2008) conducted a literature review on the survival rates of very preterm infants to determine the most common gestational age and weight for viability. Overall, neonates born under twenty-three weeks were consistently unable to survive even with intensive care. This indicates that both the twenty and twenty-four-week parameters are inconsistent with current data and cannot be defined as universal guidelines for viability.

Regardless of which study is biomedically correct in terminology and facts, the language and information presented is completely different from what women commonly use to describe their experiences. The conflict in the medical community focuses on the state of viability between twenty and twenty-four weeks, which indirectly sets twenty weeks as the absolute minimum gestational age for a stillbirth classification. As a result, any involuntary pregnancy loss before that limit will without a doubt be medically listed as a miscarriage.

The women I talked to painted a very different picture. If Lisa's description of a miscarriage as *"you're eight weeks and all of a sudden you get your period"* is universally consistent, then the cultural definition of miscarriage has a very different time limit than the medical one. The problem occurs when the cultural treatment for involuntary pregnancy loss relies upon the medical definition and guidelines. Look at Jenni's experience: *"They washed the baby and they dressed her and they wrapped her in a blanket and they gave her a little hat and they wheeled her in on a cart"* is not a medically necessary protocol. It is a cultural ritual of "you have had a baby" that follows medical guidelines. If it followed cultural ones, chances are that Lisa would have had the same experience as Jenni.

Pregnancies are medically validated when they reach twenty weeks. They are culturally validated when the mother expects that her pregnancy will definitely result in a child. In the case of the twenty-week wall, what does validation even mean? In pregnancy, the term implies that one is no longer in a static state; you are not just pregnant, you are also going to be a mother. One possible explanation of this answer lies in Lexi's narrative of how her perceptions of pregnancy changed once she felt fetal movement. This physical realization that enough time had passed for the fetus to differentiate itself from her body allowed her to accept that she was not only pregnant, but that she would possibly be having a child.

12 weeks and you're safe: the first trimester rule

Generally, women consider their pregnancies to be successful once they pass the 12-week mark. For Lisa, Amy and Jenn, who lost pregnancies after the first trimester, the invalidation of general knowledge took them by surprise:

I am devastated because I wanted children my whole life and I'd been trying for three years...While I had problems getting pregnant, [I thought] 'that's behind me now I don't have to worry about it. It's not like I'm going to have problems keeping the baby.' And when you talk about a pregnancy loss I would always consider it as commonplace to lose a pregnancy in the first trimester...but to lose it so late in the pregnancy...it's unheard of. **Lisa**

What was really horrible about the second one was I had just started telling people before it happened...We felt like we were finally in the clear...And I really felt that loss so strongly and it was so far along in the pregnancy and it just...We were really starting to feel like we were going to be fine. **Amy**

...But then the second one. I was at work...and I started bleeding and I just...that one really upset me because I felt like 'okay, I'm right, I'm about to start my second trimester and that means smooth sailing from here on' because...I think that the general common knowledge is that if you make it through the [first] trimester you're pretty much going to...that was the one that took me by surprise because that was later. **Amy**

For the women I interviewed who went on to experience another pregnancy after loss, assumptions that one was in the clear after the first trimester seemed to be thrown right out the window. A constant level of anxiety and caution infused itself within their experience, perceptions of what pregnancy is, and even the relationship that they formed with their future child:

I was completely...panic stricken the entire pregnancy. And there were a lot of people who are nervous in the first trimester. I was extremely nervous...it was just a constant...sense of just panic and fear. **Lisa**

I would say that those losses made me more aware of how tenuous pregnancy can be. I think I spent the first oh, I would say the first seventeen or eighteen weeks of my pregnancy just waiting for things to end. Just pretty sure that if things didn't end today they just might end tomorrow. And that is the worst, most horrible way to spend seventeen weeks. I was really, really anxious; very, very anxious and very sad a lot of the time...Processing most of the pregnancy that I had lost sort of later and thinking that you know during the middle of this, during the first trimester of this third pregnancy. I...had passed the due date of my second pregnancy and I would have had a three moth old after my 1st and I was really doing a lot of number games in my head and where my other pregnancies would have been at this point and not really latching on very...very tightly to the concept of this baby. I think in many ways I have...spent a lot of time...analyzing and thinking... this baby has been more like a concept for a very long time than an actual baby and it's going to be born in a very short amount of time. So that has sort of left me derailed. And once I was able to feel fetal movement for the first time, it sort of changed everything. Where in fact I was actually pregnant with an actual baby and we were going to actually be parents. Like, on a date on a calendar if all things went well. **Lexi**

Why do women assume that they are in the clear after twelve weeks? Statistically, one could answer that they are. After all, scientific studies have consistently shown that up to 80 percent of miscarriages occur in the first trimester (Abboud and Liamputtong, 2003). In describing the "survival" rate of pregnancies, Danforth's Obstetrics and Gynecology (1999) states: "More than 95 percent of pregnancies continue if a live embryo is demonstrated ultrasonically at eight weeks gestation. These embryos have a very low mortality rate during the next few weeks and the subsequent pregnancy loss rate is only 1 percent if a live fetus is seen at fourteen to sixteen weeks' gestation" (145).

All of these statistics imply that any loss after twelve weeks is extremely rare. However, if this is the case why is it that several of women I talked to experienced second trimester losses? It is possible that the length of gestation at time of loss affects how strongly the woman is impacted. If this is correct, a woman who had a significant later loss might be more inclined to share her story than someone who had an earlier loss and was not as affected. However, a review of the research on this theory found inconclusive and contradictory results (Klier et al., 2002). Another possible answer to this question lies in the time between the occurrence and the discovery of a loss. Michel and Tiu (2007) cite findings that most miscarriages in the thirteenth and fourteenth week of gestation are actually losses that occurred before twelve weeks. With this in mind, it would be safer to assume that although most losses occur in the first trimester, they may not become evident until after one thinks they are "in the clear". It would also explain what seems like a higher rate of miscarriages in the thirteenth and fourteenth week compared to the statistical rate of loss in the second trimester.

Statistics and rates medically answer the question of why women assume that they are in the clear after twelve weeks, but what about the cultural reasons? The fact that the woman starts to actually look pregnant after the first trimester may be one answer, as visibility is a key aspect of validation. The absence of noticeable physical changes in the first twelve weeks may serve as a reminder that the pregnancy is still only a possibility. Once the second trimester starts, rapidly increasing physical changes signify that the pregnancy is a concrete entity to both the woman and those around her. Community recognition affirms the confidence that the pregnancy will work out.

For women with a history of miscarriage, their risk of loss during a subsequent pregnant increases. Rai and Regan (2006) found that, "Both retrospective and prospective studies have shown that the risk of a further miscarriage increases after each successive pregnancy loss, reaching 45 percent after three consecutive pregnancy losses" (607). The awareness of a higher risk of loss combined with the memory of a past miscarriage shifts the phase of acceptance. Instead of being confident after the first twelve weeks, many of the women took much longer to feel confident if they did at all. For example, instead of assuming that her current pregnancy would be fine after the first trimester, Lexi *"spent the first oh, I would say the first seventeen or eighteen weeks of my pregnancy just waiting for things to end"*. The same is true for Lisa. Going into her pregnancy that ended in loss, her mindset had been one of *"now I don't have to worry about it, it's not like I'm going to have problems keeping the baby"*. The next time, however, she was *"panic stricken the entire pregnancy."* In terms of confidence, statistics simply can't compare to past experience.

The difference between early and later losses

I received mixed answers to whether or not gestational age at the time of loss influences the impact on the woman. For the purposes of this discussion, early loss will be defined as a loss within the first trimester and a later loss will be defined as a lost between twelve and twenty weeks gestation. For someone like Jenn, who experienced both early and late losses:

The loss when it was still fairly early in the pregnancy…I know it's hard all the way around but I would much rather, during a miscarriage, lose it early than to lose it late. **Jenn**

The difference in reactions towards losses that were early was very evident in situations of five to six week losses. According to Danforth's Obstetrics and Gynecology (1999), the first five weeks of pregnancy are defined as "the pre-embryonic period" (143), the sixth through ninth weeks of pregnancy are known as the "embryonic period", and the tenth week until the pregnancy reaches term is known as the "fetal period" (143). These losses, often termed "chemical pregnancies", would therefore occur before the fetal stage and not count as a medically legitimate pregnancy. For example, in discussing the rate of miscarriage, one study found that the risk of loss is "about 10 to 20 percent of all recognized pregnancies and 30 to 40 percent of all conceptions" (Michels and Tiu, 2007). When I asked Lisa how she was affected by her "chemical pregnancy" after her almost twenty week loss she responded:

…It barely had an impact at all actually because it was like I was pregnant for like a day. **Lisa**

Other women struggle with that general consensus that an early loss doesn't count, because for them it does:

After my second pregnancy I had a series of 'chemical pregnancies' over nearly two years. Basically, I would get pregnant, do a urine or blood test and within a week the numbers would drop and the pregnancy would end before it could really get started. Since none of these were viewed on ultrasound they weren't considered a 'clinical pregnancy' and I was told they 'don't count'. Having so many short pregnancies and the hormone roller coaster they entailed made it hard to believe I would ever get pregnant again and stay that way for more than six weeks. But I did get pregnant again about a year ago, it lasted long enough to show a heartbeat on Ultrasound but when I went for a follow up ultrasound there was no heartbeat and I was back to the usual heartbreak. **Shannon**

As miscarriage affects each woman differently, comparing early losses to later losses as general entities unfairly homogenizes the experience. There is no way to definitively answer whether or not early and later losses have the same impact. It is possible, however, to compare and contrast the different aspects that are characteristic of each situation.

The cause of approximately 50 percent of miscarriages is unknown (Neugebauer, 1996). However, the chance that the loss is a result of a chromosomal abnormality is highest during early pregnancy and decreases over time (Scott [ed.], 1999). Danforth's Obstetrics and Gynecology (1999) compared 3040 known chromosomally abnormal losses to find which stage of gestation had the highest rate of occurrence. Approximately 60 percent of these losses occurred at eight to twelve weeks, and the rate dropped to 7 percent of losses at twenty-four weeks. These results show that the majority of early pregnancy losses are an outcome of a genetic defect. They also imply that the majority of later losses are a result of a situation (such as a cord prolapse or a premature rupture of membranes) where the woman's body and not the fetus was the cause. These women have to deal both with a lost pregnancy and the possibility that their body lost it. It is much easier to say that "what happened was meant to be" if there is a genetic abnormality and the fetus would never have survived anyway. When it is a direct result of an occurrence in the woman's body, the loss becomes much more embedded with ideas of bad luck, unjustified loss, and the possibility that the outcome could have been different.

Early and late losses are also different in terms of possibility and past. Whereas early losses might come with a mourning of the pregnancy to come, later losses are additionally comprised of mourning the pregnancy that was. This includes pregnancy milestones (such as the twelve week mark), the visibility of the significant bodily changes that occur in the second trimester, and the certain awareness of the community about a possible future birth. Women with later losses may have more to mourn, but they also have more to mourn with. Other than the miscarriage, the scarcity of visual evidence means the pregnancy has not yet been

48

validated within the community. This lack of visibility also means a lack of condolence. Women may be told their early losses don't count. For some women, like Lisa, they don't. But for others, like Shannon, they do.

The proximity of the loss date with other significant dates

Dates were very important to the women that I talked to. Although I had guessed this before I started my interviews, as more stories were told I noticed an unusual trend. Several women correlated their losses with holidays and other significant events in their life:

> And I just remember feeling just…that it was just awful and it was physically and emotionally really painful and just…really devastating and it was on my mothers birthday too. And I felt weird, coincidence you know the first miscarriage was on a holiday and the second one was on my mother's birthday…**Amy**

> My first pregnancy ended in miscarriage on Thanksgiving of last year. And my second miscarriage happened on Easter of last year. **Lexi**

> The next one was a miscarriage and that was in…February of 95…excuse me, I'm sorry. March. St. Patrick's day, how could I forget that? … He [her husband] was wary because his father had died on St. Patrick's Day when he was like 5 years old. **Cindy**

The occurrence of losses on significant dates is interesting, but what is fascinating is why the women describe their losses in these terms. It is possible that a correlation to universally important and acknowledged dates allows others a way to find personal significance in the loss. For the woman, who may not be able to present physical evidence of what occurred, this could be a way to shift the loss from a personal experience to something that existed in the real world. A date implies that something happened, but an important date implies that it was significant. In acknowledging the loss through what others perceive to be meaningful, women are able to create a much more concrete awareness of the miscarriage.

Correlation between significance of loss and the length of time since the event

When writing up the questions for my interviews I almost omitted ones whose answers seemed obvious. Of course involuntary pregnancy loss was significant in a woman's life. I was quite wrong in this assumption. For some it was and for some it wasn't. For some, time had changed their answer:

I don't think about them every day…you know it's been five years, well almost six years now actually. But you know I thought of it when I found out I was pregnant. Things like that. When it does come up, you know. It's kind of a sad memory and everything but I'm kind of at the point now where I've just kind of moved on from it I guess. I don't dwell on it really. **Amber**

Yeah. And I think that I always will but I can also imagine that in fifteen years I might give a different answer. It still feels like a new thing that has happened so it feels significant. **Jenni**

At the time, yes. But right now, twenty-two years later, twenty-one years later, nineteen years later. Not as much. **Amy**

Yeah, I think it's significant. I actually don't think about it very much. When I read over your questions…I started to maybe relive parts of it that I hadn't for a while…[It's] sort of deeper but it's always there so I can call on the feelings at any time. **Kirsten**

No, because I have other kids to take care of. It was significant but over the years, you know, it tends to get less and less. It's not that I don't think about it because I do. You know, and it's like 'okay I have kids that would be…eleven, twelve, I would have had one that would be fifteen'. And you know when the birthday time comes around…I always remember them. **Cindy**

When reading these responses it is important to understand that for Jenni, Amy, Kirsten, and Cindy the pregnancy loss itself was a significant event. However, as time passed it integrated itself into their life. Cindy and Kirsten's comments that their losses are still thought about imply that the event has retained importance over time. However, it no longer supersedes other significant moments in their history and present life.

In addition to time, whether or not the women currently had children seemed to make a difference in the significance of the loss. Amy, Kirsten, and Cindy currently have children. For Shannon, who does not:

> Yes, it's changed everything about me, how I feel about my life and my family, how my career has changed. **Shannon**

The experience is also significant for Jenni. However, I think it is important to note Jenni's remark *"but I can also imagine that in like fifteen years I might give a different answer"*. Time might change her response. The question is whether she defines such an interval as the passing of days or the possibility of having a child.

Age of the woman at the time of pregnancy

Age plays a very interesting role in pregnancy. There seems to be a significant reaction to a pregnant woman if her age does not fall into what is considered the normal age range to have a child (Early twenty's until age thirty-five) and where pregnancy most often occurs (Scott [ed.], 1999). However this concept of a childbearing age range as a homogenous group could very quickly become problematic. For example, a woman who is twenty and experiences a pregnancy loss may have a very different reaction than a woman who is forty. With that understanding in mind I asked all of the women if and how their age affected their experience with pregnancy loss. Quite a few were unable to answer the question. Some felt that being older made the situation better as a result of gained experience. Cindy, who is currently fifty-three and experienced a loss at thirty-seven, responded:

> Oh let's see… I think I was probably more able to handle it, you know? And then, I wasn't totally naïve as far as…the possibility of what could happen. **Cindy**

Others felt that youth would have helped them in terms of time left to try again. Jenni, who was also thirty-seven when she experienced a loss, responded:

> A lot and actually that was another one of those things that

hit me almost immediately when it happened. I was like 'god I wish I was ten years younger' because here I was at thirty-seven...you know and at thirty-seven, you're already on the wrong side. I was already on the wrong side of thirty-five. And I kind of knew that my heart and my body were both going to need a lot of time to recuperate and recoup and reset. And by the time we were trying again I would be closer to forty than I was to thirty-five, which was true. It sucks that it happened so early in our marriage and I don't wish losses on anyone, but I wish this had happened to someone who was ten years younger than me, because then they have a much better chance, not of ever replacing that baby but of eventually having a successful pregnancy, which is in part a healing experience. So I'm very aware of the fact that this may be completely out of reach for me. **Jenni**

Milestones are very important aspects of pregnancy. However, are they important in themselves or as a result of the significance we give it? Perhaps the best way to understand such a theme is to explore how timing is beneficial and what parties are affected by their influence.

For pregnancy, milestones such as timing are integral to the validation of what is becoming, and in the case of miscarriage, what would have been. Rather than one specific aspect, validation encompasses the different ways in which pregnancy is acknowledged and legitimized. For the medical community, pregnancy is confirmed when the fetus is detected by ultrasound at approximately five weeks (Scott [ed], 1999). In society, pregnancy is acknowledged when the woman's significantly larger "belly" announces it. Most importantly, the woman experiences specific occurrences that lead to the acceptance of her pregnancy.

The act of growing a human being is an incredible physical and mental shift. In order to accept that the body contains an entity that it grows into a human, the mind must go through a series of significant phases. At first, women do not perceive themselves as pregnant. Rather, pregnancy is a separate event that is occurring within their body and is not a baby (Sonstegard, 1983). In order to begin planning for a child, the pregnant woman needs to shift her perception of pregnancy from that of a separate event in her body to a phase of herself. Although acceptance of pregnancy involves the merging of a body and situation, the ability to conceptualize the idea of a baby occurs when the fetus is viewed as a separate entity within the woman's body (Sonstegard, 1983).

Studies (Adolfsson et al, 2004; Wright, 2010) have attempted to track the phases of pregnancy and the point at which it is validated. In the first phase of Wright's (2010) study, *Experiencing the Pregnancy*, the women found out about the pregnancy, developed a relationship that started at the moment of conception, continued to develop this bond through preparation for the baby, and experienced a gradual personality shift to "mothering" (taking care of the potential child) with an emphasis on individual responsibility. Like Wright, Adolfsson et al. (2004) also identified a time interval between a woman finding out that she is pregnant and the point at which she accepts it and begins to plan and anticipate a child.

Milestones are the system by which we try to keep track of these changes. It benefits some by validating their pregnancy, and conceals those to whom it has not. When a miscarriage occurs, it affects how important the loss is perceived to be. In the absence of the visibility of the fetus, time actually serves as a substitute marker for the physical entity to be mourned. When someone says that they have lost a pregnancy at nineteen weeks, it is the number that allows us to put that experience in perspective.

Power

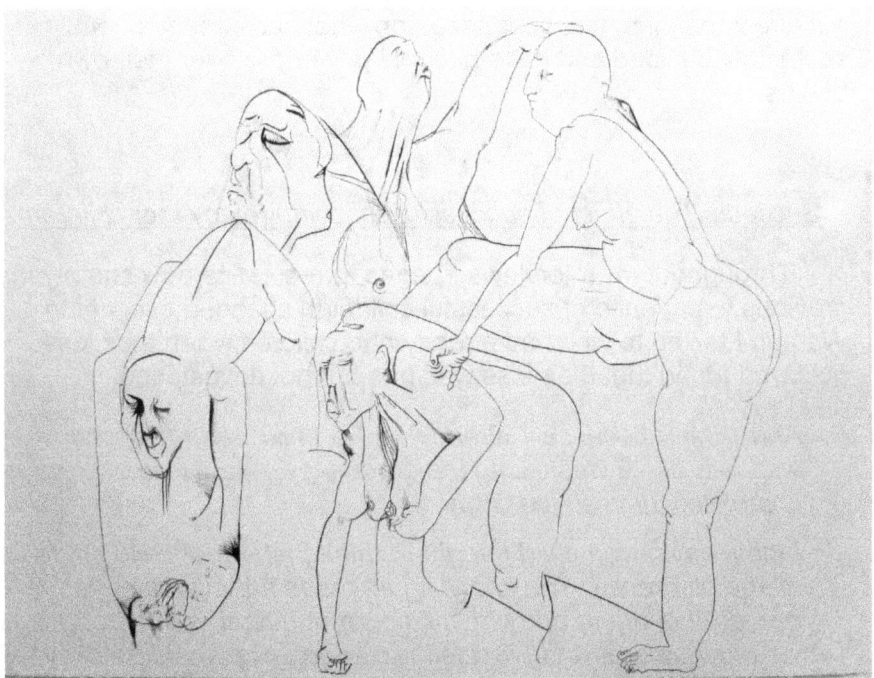

     If pregnancy is a state of change in one's body, miscarriage represents an inability to control it. The need to personally determine if and when you have children appeared again and again in many of the topics discussed during my interviews. These factors serve as a foundation for various emotions that the women I talked to experienced during their losses.

     Power encompasses many things. For example, *success* is reflected in holding power, whereas already having living children is seen as successful and mediates some of the loss of power that can occur during miscarriage. Another component is *hope*, the internal drive to gain and sustain power. This appears in the decision of whether or not to try again after a loss. *Chances*, the limited amount of times it is possible to gain power before it dissipates, happens every time a woman attempts fertility treatments such as In Vitro Fertilization (IVF). There is also the power of *intention*, which is a mindset that mental willpower can influence bodily events. This action is evident in a woman's mental attempt to stop an involuntary pregnancy loss. *Powerlessness*, the forfeiture of these attempts, is a state of no control. It is here that one must acknowledge that they have had no success, have lost hope, have run out of chances, can not direct their intentions, cannot stop what has already been seemingly decided and have become powerless over their own bodies.

Success: The effect of successful childbirth (aka: other children)

Throughout my interviews I began to recognize how sharply the previous experience of successful childbirth changed everything. Women I talked to who had already had children when their loss occurred found that their loss was bad but not devastating:

> And I think because I already had a child...and that one, it was only like 9 weeks into the pregnancy. Again I wasn't...so completely devastated. **Amy**

> I think having...a child (laughs) I think that a real child made all the difference. You know, it just made me think that yes, I can do this again and we will figure out what went wrong if we did it before. And I just felt like everything would be okay. **Amy**

> ...[During] the second pregnancy loss...I just felt like [I wanted] the more natural approach. I don't know if it was because I had another baby already [and] I didn't really feel ready for another, but it wasn't as bad for me. **Kirsten**

Although having previous children seemed to significantly help women get through the involuntary pregnancy loss, the possibility of future children was a bit more conflicted. Lisa went on to have another child after her loss and felt that it really helped her:

> The only thing that helps me through it is to know that...if I had had her I don't know what would have happened, but I

*wouldn't have the one I have now. **Lisa***

However, before she had her daughter the idea of focusing on trying to have another child created a serious conflict of replacement:

*You know and then, not just my friends but everybody who knew or everybody who found out, they just didn't understand. Because they were like 'oh you can have another one'. But they didn't understand that it had nothing to do with that. First of all I didn't know if I could have another one and second of all, it wasn't just like this thing...you know, it was my hopes and dreams. It was just...it was my daughter. **Lisa***

This sentiment was also strongly felt by Shannon, who has experienced multiple losses but not a live birth:

*I hated when people told me 'you're still young'. Like the babies that died didn't matter because I had plenty of time to have more. Anything that invalidates or denies their existence is a major blow to me. **Shannon***

Part of the reason for the conflict surrounding "having another one" is that Shannon and Lisa were not sure if they even **could**. This doubt goes against the cultural assumption and expectation that a baby is always the result of a pregnancy. A lot of the women I talked to had been very aware of this idea:

*And I bled for most of the pregnancy because of the polyp so I didn't have...I never really had the experience of like 'I'm pregnant and I'm sure that there's going to be a baby at the end of this' because it was...there was never a point where my body felt like it had really stabilized with the pregnancy. So I think that's one of the ways in which my experience is different from the other stories I've heard where people are just like really hopeful and it was going to be totally normal...It's...you're totally devastated. There's a way in which we were prepared for the possibility that this wasn't going to work out. But we were not ever in a million years prepared for the possibility that we were going to deliver a baby at twenty weeks because you can't get ready for that basically. **Jenni***

The women were not the only ones affected by such assumptions. Partners, such as Jenni's husband, also found themselves surprised by the loss:

Being a dad is a huge part of his identity. And this was just such a massive blow. He is generally more optimistic person than I am and he really, really believed that the pregnancy was going to work and that the baby was going to be fine. During all those times when I never could get really to allow myself to think that or when I was very aware of the problems. So he was…you know, it was terrible. It was really terrible for him. **Jenni**

After experiencing a loss, interacting with others who still fully expect their pregnancies to work out also created a source of conflict:

Since my losses I can't help but notice how women I know blithely announce their pregnancies with such assurance that in nine months they will have their baby. I can't congratulate them on getting pregnant. I know it's difficult for many but since I've done it so many times I don't feel that way for myself. I think 'good luck' instead of 'congratulations'. **Shannon**

   In order to understand why previous successful childbirth played such a significant role in how the women I interviewed perceived the magnitude of their loss, the role of raising children must be addressed. If womanhood is defined by motherhood in our society, then pregnancy can be seen as the rite of passage wherein a female assumes her role as a woman. Rich (1976) describes this use of pregnancy to join the community in reflecting: "I only know that to have a child was to assume adult womanhood to the full, to prove myself to be 'like other women" (25). The women I interviewed who had already experienced successful childbirth have been initiated into our society as mothers. Their loss was bad but not devastating because they had already proven that they could reproductively succeed. In comparison, women without children who miscarry lose both the pregnancy and the chance of social initiation. Pregnancy loss disrupts the "rite of passage" and halts the transition from nulliparity to motherhood. As there are no protocols for this situation the woman is caught without a way to be initiated back into the community (Layne, 2003).

After listening to the women's stories, I disagree with Layne's (2003) statement. There is a way to be reinitiated back into society; through a successful childbirth. This protocol is evident in Lisa's story. She was frustrated when those around her mentioned that she could have another because *"First of all I didn't know if I could have another one"*. At this point, she had left her position as a woman who has never been pregnant but had failed to reach the initiation point of becoming a mother. However, this changed once she had her daughter and she was able to claim the title of that role.

But what happens when multiple attempts still leave you without success? It is a very hard thing to not be able to succeed while others seem to have no problem. As McCracken (2008) mentioned in her memoir, "Still, I wouldn't have minded a pause in the whole business. A sudden harmless moratorium on babies being born" (43). This sentiment echoes Shannon's frustration with women who approach pregnancy with complete confidence of succeeding. But wishing women good luck instead of congratulations, pregnancy becomes a game of chance. Unfortunately, the greater the risk, the greater the reward of success.

Hope: Deciding to try again

The theme of hope came up when the women I interviewed discussed their decisions to try again or to give up. Some of them felt torn between their need for children and their capacity to withstand another loss:

Yes, I wonder if I should give up. I tell myself when I'm going through the agony of another miscarriage that this has to be the last time. But then some time goes by and I think about trying again. I can't give up on the chance that it might work out. I don't want to give up on the possibility that I could have biological children with my husband. **Shannon**

I would like to have more children still, but then there are losses. And the risk. When you get pregnant again and you don't know how many miscarriages you'll ever have. But I do want more. More children. **Jenn**

For women like Lisa who now have a child, the choice can also weigh on whether or not another pregnancy would even be beneficial to their current family structure:

> *I mean just… we have one more embryo…[we are] trying to decide what to do with it. I feel compelled to use it but I don't really want to go through this again…I am so…I can't tell you. I don't know if you have children, but this is the most amazing thing in the world that happens, this baby. And I wanted to put all my attention into her and I can't imagine dividing my attention. Even though I wanted twins all along and I wanted more than one child I just cant imagine doing that at this point. You know, that coupled with the experience of having to go through a pregnancy again. So I don't know. I probably…like I said I feel compelled to use the embryo because I just can't imagine what to do with one surviving embryo. I just can't imagine destroying it.* **Lisa**

For Susan, the conflict lay not in her decision to give up trying but in finding a space where she wouldn't feel out of place as a result of her choice:

> *I did go to a couple SHARE meetings…and I went to the one at [the local hospital] that [the facilitator] runs which is a great group. But I didn't really continue going because most of the people in the group I think have had bigger pregnancy losses and a lot of those are still in that mode of trying to have another baby. And…a couple people even said…I can try again. I needed to…I was different from that. I wasn't there. Resolving that.* **Susan**

The conflict between the need for family and the capacity for loss depends on the strength and history of each side. Need is a reflection on what one does not have, and capacity is a measurement of how much one can have. For the women I talked to, need depended on how many children the woman currently had, how badly the woman wanted to raise a child, how important the role of raising children was culturally, and what would be lost if there were none. Capacity depended on how many losses the woman had experienced, how they had impacted the woman, the strength and size of her support system and her level of resilience.

For someone like Shannon, her need for children encompassed the fact that she had never experienced a successful birth, that she wanted a child seemingly more than anything else and that not having a child would be significantly detrimental to her mental health. Her capacity for loss encompassed her multiple losses, the significantly negative impact the losses had on her relationships, the lack of support she felt during previous experiences and her level of physical and mental exhaustion.

In contrast, Jenn's need for children encompassed the fact that she had gone through several successful childbirths, that she still wanted more children, and that she grew up in a culture that promoted a large family (she has sixteen siblings). On the other side of the debate, Jenn's capacity for loss encompassed her multiple losses, the negative impact that her later loss had on her, the strong church community that supported her during previous losses, and how quickly she was able to move forward after her experiences.

In spite of the risk of additional loss, many women do try to have a successful birth after a miscarriage. Although this can be considered positive in terms of the overall resiliency of the involuntary pregnancy loss community, what about women who can't? The choice may seem individual, but the reality may be universal. As a result of no longer trying to become pregnant, Susan did not fit into the available pregnancy loss support structure. Perhaps the decision to keep trying involves not just the need for children and the capacity for loss, but also the risk of not fitting into the parameters of either community.

Chances: In Vivo Veritas, In Vitro Maybe

Within the active state of hope is the mental perception of chance. This theme popped up quite a bit when women talked about their attempts to get pregnant. Several of the women I interviewed had undergone or were currently undergoing Assisted Reproductive Technology (ART). This umbrella term for fertility treatment includes many different procedures. The two main treatments that the women used were: in vitro fertilization (IVF), the process of creating an embryo outside of the body and transferring it to the uterus; and Intrauterine Insemination (IUI) (Scott [ed], 1999). ART procedures are very expensive and most women can only afford so many cycles. The limited amount of chances available and the challenge of becoming pregnant became a large part of these women's stories:

So I'd been trying for three years before I got pregnant, in vitro and insemination. We got pregnant using IUI, which is an insemination with fertility drugs. **Lisa**

My husband and I had been trying IVF for four years. And we went through fertility treatment; we went through IUI, and then IVF. And ...in IVF...so we had a good cycle but I had a third embryo... And at that point I had given up hope, I felt like, 'whatever'. **Susan**

We've actually been trying to get pregnant for over a year and...we've done a couple or rounds of fertility treatments. Not full IVF but some fertility drugs and we haven't had any luck so right now we're getting insurance clearance to get a couple of rounds of IVF and see what happens. **Jenni**

Fertility treatments seemed to take a large toll on the women and created a stronger focus on getting pregnant rather than on the pregnancy itself. IVF may change both how women get pregnant as well as how it is even confirmed:

I had ...in vitro and [on] my first [cycle] I got the pregnancy result and it was great. Then you have to get a bunch of blood tests. It's not just 'oh I'm pregnant'; you keep getting these blood tests. I got the first blood test and everything was great. And then they were like 'okay you should double within two days', but it didn't double. So it was like well 'we don't want to get worried but it didn't double' so I'm like 'okay great', you know? And then it was fine from then on and just doubled and doubled and was okay... So then it was like all things leading up to the ultrasound to see if there was actually anything there. It looked at that moment like there had been one [embryo], one had taken and the other didn't look like it had taken. And then we went back to confirm that there was just one, one pregnancy. **Lisa**

For some of the women the availability of IVF and medical treatment depended on their insurance. This shifted a lot of the control from the women to another source and created a limited number of chances to try again:

The doctors are already making an effort to find out if there is anything like, 'what can they test me for?' So...there have been times when it's been like 'well we think you really need this test but we don't think insurance will cover you'. Which is a pretty normal thing for people to hear but it's really amped up for me because it's like 'Oh my god if I don't get this test does it mean that my baby will die?' You know? So it goes to this kind of stratospheric level. **Susan**

For Susan, insurance will no longer cover fertility treatments because of her age. Her story is a good example of what happens when chances run out:

The first thing is to just say all right. And I didn't expect it to hit me so hard and it did. And I think too that if I had had other chances. Like I didn't have any other chances you know? That was it. I mean I was at the age where insurance…we could have paid for ourselves but it's like we couldn't afford it. **Susan**

Many assume that chances to have a successful birth only occur during pregnancy. But what about the energy needed to even reach that point? For a woman who struggles with infertility, her efforts to conceive often overshadow the energy needed for confidence in pregnancy. Procedures such as In Vitro Fertilization are extremely expensive, invasive, promise no definite result, and serve as a constant reminder that the woman cannot become pregnant on her own (Scott [ed.], 1999).

What happens when a woman does successfully become pregnant through ART? There is a general assumption that fertility treatments put the woman at a higher risk for a miscarriage. However, this aspect of ART does not limit the number of opportunities the woman has. Schieve et al. (2003) analyzed 62,228 pregnancies and found no significant correlation between pregnancies resulting from these technologies and an increased risk of miscarriage. In fact:

"The spontaneous abortion (miscarriage) rate for this US population-based sample of ART pregnancies was comparable to rates previously reported for naturally conceived clinical pregnancies…" (963). Although it is encouraging that women who use ART may not have higher rates of loss, results such as these should not discount the valid possibility of miscarriage. In contrast to women who conceived naturally, women who become pregnant through ART and then lose a pregnancy must also mourn the lengthy process it took to even get to that point.

With ART and especially IVF, the number of attempts a woman can try directly correlates with her material assets and capacity for physical and emotional stress. Financial limitations are a main factor in the number of chances allotted for conception. For example, in 2006 one cycle of in vitro fertilization cost approximately $12,513, and the average total cost per live birth was $41,132 (Chambers et al., 2009). Levy and Widra (2001) also cited studies that priced a successful treatment of IVF at $50,000 to $100,000.

Insurance covered IVF for several of the women I talked to. However, policies have set limitations on the number of cycles allowed. After that, treatments must be paid completely out of pocket. When insurance denies coverage and effectively cuts off any viable future attempts to become pregnant, it is almost as if the woman is being punished for ruining her chance. She had it and she failed. Susan is a perfect example of how finances and insurance limited her chances to the point that she no longer had any. She is also an example of how age counts. After her pregnancy loss, she tried to go through one more cycle of IVF. However, *"After forty-three once you have three cycles they don't let you have any more treatment because it is no longer a fertility factor"*.

The physical and emotional toll that these treatments take on the women also limits the number of tries available. As is evident through Lisa's story, going through a cycle of IVF includes constant blood draws and ultrasounds. What she didn't mention was "the identification of risk factors through an in-depth, tailored history and physical, as well as testing to document ovulation, possible postcoital test, hysterosalpingogram, semen analysis, possible laparascopy..." (Scott [ed], 1999:245). There is only so much a body can take. The number of times one is willing to show up and sit through test after test determines how likely one is to gain or forever lose the chance for successful childbirth.

The Power of Intention: body over mind

In describing their reactions to realizing that they were going to be experiencing an involuntary pregnancy loss many women mentioned how they mentally tried to stop what was happening:

I just remember lying on my back in my office at work. Just, just thinking, 'Oh I hope this isn't happening, I hope this isn't happening, I can't believe this is happening'. **Amy**

Kirsten tried to deny what she was seeing in hopes that it would not be true:

I didn't really believe the doctor when he said it was a miscarriage and not a pregnancy. So he did a vaginal ultrasound, I guess to convince me. I still didn't, it wasn't real to me. So, I sort of expected to not bleed and just to show that I was not as far along as we thought so therefore they would see what they thought they needed to see. You know, there wouldn't be a heartbeat because there wasn't a heart yet and that I was still pregnant. So when I started to bleed...the doctor...recommended a dilation and curettage. And I, I went ahead with it. They did it under general anesthesia... And I probably, I wish that I hadn't done that because it seemed like what they did was take the pregnancy away. I mean it's ridiculous. I know I was bleeding, and I had lots of clumps of tissue that I had collected for the doctor to do tests on. So I should have believed him but it still seemed like if I hadn't gone and allowed them to do that maybe I'd still be pregnant. It just kind of felt like I had something taken away from me. **Kirsten**

Other women, such as Amy, remember bargaining with a greater force in order to have a successful pregnancy:

You know I always stop myself and I think "I remember saying to myself if 'I could just have a kid and it just works out I will just be the best mother and I'll never take it for granted just how precious they are to me'. And so I still think about that. **Amy**

The power of intention has woven itself into women's stories. The belief that the mind physically controls the body may stem from societal perceptions of dualism. This concept is based on the theory that an individual "is a single person with both body and thought so related by nature that the thought can move the body and feel the things which happen to it" (Cottingham, 1993:126). If the mind can

64

cause physical changes in the body, then theoretically it should be able to stop it from losing a pregnancy.

Assumptions that such control exists are evident in society's perception of how much the woman regulates her reproduction. In her analysis of motherhood as a continuation of patriarchy, Rich (1976) found that "the power of the mother is, first of all, to give or withhold...nowhere else...does a woman possess such literal power over life and death" (68). As a result of this power, there is a very clear cultural understanding that birth will always be the "inevitable expectation of pregnancy" (Layne, 2003:72).

However, when Amy was lying on the floor of her office thinking, *"Oh I hope this isn't happening, I hope this isn't happening, I can't believe this is happening"*, the power of intention did not work. When Kirsten denied her ultrasound results and *"sort of expected to not bleed"*, her mind could not stop her body. No matter how hard we try, "I think, therefore I am" does not translate into "I'm pregnant, therefore I am going to have a baby."

When the power of the self did not work, some of the women turned to another form of intention: bargaining. Amy remembers promising that if she were granted a child, she would be the best mother. For this to work, another entity would have to be in control of the pregnancy. If this is the case, the power of intention may exist, but we are not the ones who control it.

Powerlessness: loss of control

For a lot of the women, the power of intention gradually gave way to a feeling of powerlessness and an acknowledgement that there was nothing to be done:

> *I know they feel a little bit powerless to help and there's a way in which that's just true. There is an unhelpful aspect of this.* **Jenn**

With Amy, the loss of control played a role in the level of grief that she experienced:

> *And then, it just sucks because I knew what was happening; you kind of, you've been through it once. You know they are*

65

like 'maybe it's going to be okay and maybe, you're just spotting and that happens'. But it's like, 'no, something's horribly wrong'. You have an intuition about those things I think. And it was just such a grim feeling and just the whole summer after that I think I was really depressed. **Amy**

For Susan, her acknowledgement of powerlessness did not just apply to her. It also pertained to her higher power:

I think that my job definitely...It made that a little harder, definitely a little harder in some ways. It challenged my faith a little bit because I just remember thinking 'how could God be so cruel?' It would have been better to have never gotten pregnant that to have gotten pregnant and then lose it. It's really...I remember feeling like 'how did this happen'. **Susan**

There is "a need to create a sense of cultural control over birth, a natural process resistant to control" (Layne, 2003:81). This paradox can create a strong sense of powerlessness that I found in my interviews. But what factors actually create this feeling? Is it the process of the miscarriage itself or the influence of social and cultural authority? These authorities are best explained when defined in the context of the role a healthcare provider plays. Social authority is the capacity of a provider to control access to medical interventions (Joraleman, 2010). Cultural authority is the notion that certain providers have power over others because of the respect held for their knowledge and training. When combined, these two authorities give the healthcare provider higher cultural capital and grant their decisions the right to not be questioned.

Involuntary pregnancy loss is primarily considered a medical issue, as there are possible physical complications for the woman during the experience. As a result, many women use a treatment method advised by their doctor. The language of these medical experiences may convince the woman that she is ignorant about what is occurring and produce limitations on what she feels she is allowed to do and say. For example, when asked about the treatment method for her second loss, Jenni responded:

The second one was a delivery. Or I...I don't know what else to call it I mean...medically I don't think I'm allowed to. **Jenni**

Kirsten is another example of how the power of the provider superseded her own. Through ultrasound, the doctor concluded that she was losing her pregnancy and used cultural authority to convince her that medical intervention was necessary. Surgical treatment implies that the doctor possesses the ability to complete the miscarriage because the woman can't. As Kirsten was not mentally prepared to acknowledge her pregnancy loss, she felt like she *"had something taken away from me."*

Both Jenni and Kirsten's stories illustrate how the hierarchy of power through social authority can convince an individual that they have no control and accept powerlessness. Power is intertwined with miscarriage because the experience encompasses so many aspects of life. As a result, "a woman's emotional response to pregnancy loss is more than simply personal or individual; those emotional responses are culturally, socially, and historically produced" (Reagan, 2003:373).

Pain

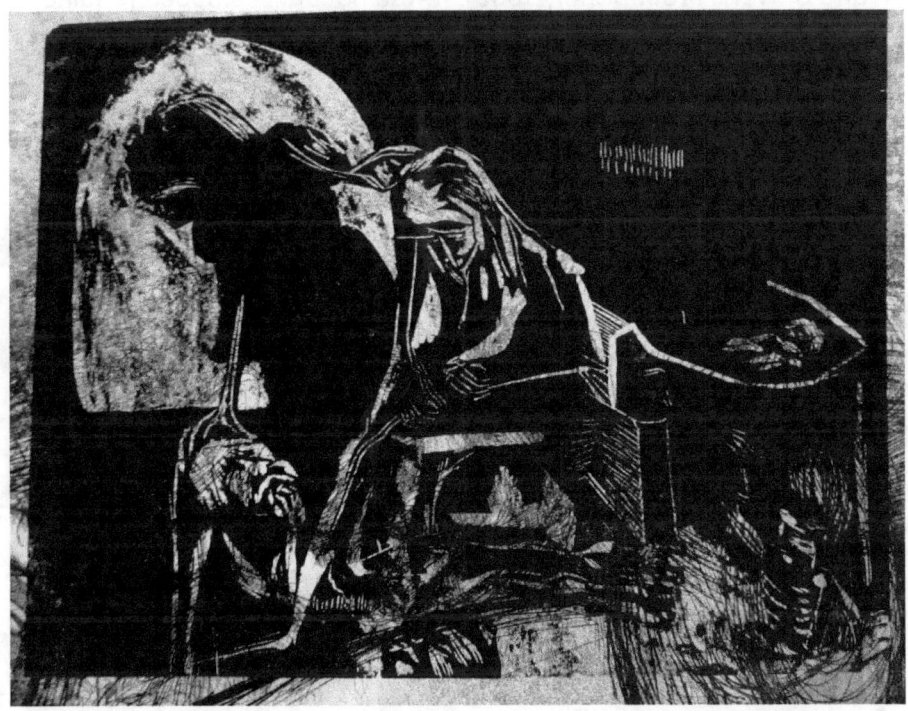

        Choosing to devote a school year to the topic and experience of involuntary pregnancy loss raised many questions from the women interviewed as well as those around me. Very few people understood why I would undertake such a subject. It appears at first glance that involuntary pregnancy loss creates one of the most basic forms of sadness. I would argue that its capabilities for pain are a combination of many different types. Through my interviews I discovered physical pain, emotional pain, the pain of isolation, the pain of seeing other pregnancies, and the impact that pain has on altering ones life and fundamental view of the world. All of these aspects and countless others combine to form the pain that we associate with involuntary pregnancy loss.

Physical Pain

Throughout my research, I constantly read about the emotional and mental turmoil that women go through during miscarriage (Abboud and Liamputtong, 2005; Adolfsson et al., 2004; Bansen and Stevens, 1992; Brier, 1999). It was not until I stopped reading texts and started talking to women that physical pain came into the dialogue. Regardless of treatment, many had vivid descriptions of what an involuntary pregnancy loss tangibly feels like:

> *I took Misoprostol instead of doing another D and C. After I had wished I had done the D and C because I felt like the Misoprostol was more traumatic than surgery. Passing the tissue was very painful even though I had Vicodin. But the worst part was waking up in the early morning hours in a drugged haze and stumbling to the toilet and to feel what I felt and look down and see what I saw. I nearly passed out, from blood loss or from the experience, I'm not sure. Somehow I managed to crawl back to bed before I fell down.* **Shannon**

> *We had been together eight years and…suddenly I had this horrific pain. And it turns out I was having a miscarriage…I mean I lived with this horrific pain thinking something was wrong and I would be in pain for hours a day. And then it would kind of subside. I went through this for about two weeks.* **Malissa**

> *It was very painful, extremely painful to go through it, the contractions. And it's shocking to see a fetus too. I buried the fetus…outside in my garden.* **Jennifer**

> *And I just remember feeling that [it] was just awful and it was physically and emotionally really painful.* **Amy**

In focusing on the emotional grief and mourning of involuntary pregnancy loss, we often forget that miscarriage actually hurts. Similar to labor, the cervix dilates and the uterus contracts painfully (Scott [ed.], 1999). These facts are often obscured by the focus on the mental experience. Reagan (2003) found that "Today, when emotional distress following miscarriage is highlighted, physical stress of the event tends to be obscured" (359).

If physical pain does not seem to exist in the information on miscarriage, its manifestations definitely don't. For example, blood is rarely talked about. With the exception of a few sentences describing its visibility as a possible symptom, one of the main physical aspects of miscarriage is not explained in detail. Although each case is different, the descriptions in the medical textbooks and literature I read seemed to heavily contrast with the women's stories I heard. For example, in describing the symptoms of a threatened miscarriage, Danforth's Obstetrics and Gynecology (1999) states: "Bleeding associated with threatened miscarriage is typically scanty..." (144). This was not the case for the beginning symptoms of Cindy's second loss:

> *My older daughter Sara was in a concert at school, so...we got there and...I was feeling all this pressure like I was about to get my period or something, you know? So we go in and we sit down in the concert hall and you know, it's the auditorium with the floor slant...All of a sudden I felt this burst of liquid and I thought 'this is weird'...and then I felt this bigger squirt, and I thought I had peed my pants or something. So I squatted down in between the seats...and then I looked down at the floor and there was just a stream of blood going down...it was just like...I couldn't stop it. It was just going. Come to find out I was having a miscarriage. So they parade me through the school like 'gush gush gush'...all the way down to where the nurse's office was...we've got this trail of blood and all these footprints...Cindy*

This experience is unique but not unusual. There is a major difference between a scanty amount of bleeding and a stream of blood. I have spent time in operating rooms observing surgical treatments for miscarriage. From those experiences I know: there is a lot of blood, and there is no way the medical community could miss that fact. Although textbooks may not give a complete picture, at least they acknowledge the presence of blood. The problem lies in the translation of that information. Pregnancy loss books written for the general public generally don't discuss these aspects. Unless a woman gains access to scientific literature, she may have no idea what a miscarriage can physically entail. That may partially explain why Shannon nearly passed out after the shock of seeing how much blood there was after her D and C. Another little talked about aspect of miscarriage is that losing a pregnancy is not just losing blood. If a woman decides to go through the experience naturally without medical treatment like Jennifer did, the sight of the fetus may also shock her.

Many argue that miscarriage is not validated as a real loss because there is no physical evidence. I would argue that there is, it's just not the kind we want. It is inappropriate to describe such an experience graphically, especially if it involves uterine blood. In her historical analysis of menstruation, Martin (2001) found that "menstrual blood, to be sure, was often seen as foul and unclean" (31). Eventually, "even the process itself is seen as a disorder" (35). If miscarriage carries similar connotations as menstruation, then blood is not the only taboo. It is also inappropriate to talk about the process, the actual physical loss and pain.

Emotional Pain: the experience of grief

A story is a story is a story in that every woman's tale is her own. Under the umbrella of emotional grief I found sadness in delayed reactions to the loss, in the instant that one realizes waiting is the only option, in the announcement of loss, in the surprise of getting through the days, in the dullness of the aftermath, and in ways that have not yet been unearthed:

*So initially it was totally like…I remember feeling sad but I just felt kind of…the thing is I had just had similar losses recently…I lost my dad that year. And a few other things that happened…I kind of I think I had more of a delayed reaction. So it was maybe a few weeks later that it really hit me and it hit me hard…and I was really depressed. And I work in an OB office…so it got be really hard to be at work sometimes. It had been a really a long day. One of the doctors asked me to go in and talk to a patient…who had just had a loss, and I just burst into tears and I was like…'I can't do it, I will get you some information, I will get you some resources'…but if I go in I'm going to start crying and that's not going to be helpful to anybody. It was just so raw you know…and it was just so hard. **Susan***

I…called my doctor and she said 'just lie down for a little while and relax'. I was on the floor and I had shut the door and I laid down on my back and…and just…I just remember the tears streaming down the sides of my face…and I was looking up at the ceiling like 'why is this happening'. **Amy**

Although you know you have these moments where you're just like 'God', you know, 'I've lost three babies'. That's just a very sad feeling when they're so wanted you know, you really, really want them and it really just tears you up. **Amy**

…My daughter was delivered early, was delivered prematurely, at nineteen weeks. And she died in childbirth. And I, I named her, her name was Sally Ann and I said that she…I gave her stats. I don't even remember them today but it was like…you know. Eight ounces and…nine inches long or whatever she was and that she was, she was absolutely perfect, and she was perfect in every way other than dead. And you know it's just something like that. It's just sadness. **Lisa**

I was pretty medicated. Actually. I had anti-anxiety pills, and they put me on an antidepressant for a little bit… I don't really feel like I've gotten over it so much as…I put my self into work. I was very emotional. I was getting into fights with my boss all the time; I was screaming or breaking down. I was really…not doing very well; I was just extremely emotional. I would get upset, you know, and start to cry over like the smallest bit of pressure. [I] just really kept myself hidden. I would come home after work and try not to fail. I tried to figure out what my next steps were. **Lisa**

I think the only thing that I might add is just that; the thing that I was unprepared for was the nature of the grieving process. And I don't know that a lot of people even notice or are aware of miscarriage before twelve weeks. People tell me about how common that is, but they don't talk about the grief associated with that. Or now and then you hear about…like preemie's who die in the NICU and you hear that it's very common but you don't; I didn't have any sense of what the grieving process is like. And I will just say that is it nothing like the five stages in my personal [opinion]. And I don't know if that is something that is particular to pregnancy loss. **Jenni**

There are days when I can really feel completely fine, and there are days when it's like absolutely being in a chokehold and there's a huge unpredictability factor with it. And lots of things can be triggering and nothing can be triggering and I think that is one of the things that lost moms go through that is hard for their communities to understand. That you can be five years out, and something can come up for you. And you can be laid out for a week. You know, at a time when people think like, 'oh but you should be better' or 'you've come to have two more children'. And that's also where...you asked the stigma question and I think that's what I'm getting at. There's a stigma in...grief. In grieving for too long. **Jenni**

And when my pregnancy ended, I think everything just kind of got very, uh, dull for a while. And I really kind of let the color drain from the world for a long time. **Lexi**

For Lexi and Malissa, who discovered they were pregnant as a result of realizing they were losing the pregnancy, grief did not have a place to rest. Both women felt that there was no time allowed for it:

And...so I asked him to check it and he said yeah. That I was passing...having a miscarriage...and by this time this was a different relationship. The third pregnancy...I didn't have any time to get all emotional now or anything like that. [It was] just so, quick and...over with. **Malissa**

And so my second pregnancy was definitely something that we unfortunately didn't know about. So I had been told to wait several months to begin trying again and my husband and I were actively not trying. And so I had had a period that lasted very, very long. Three weeks. And my acupuncturist finally cornered me and said, 'I want you to take a pregnancy test. It's really important that you do this.' And I was pregnant, and I was also miscarrying. So that was a really...confusing and disheartening and really sad time. I think I was, I definitely was not in the headspace where I had known I was pregnant; I didn't know that I was miscarrying. [There was a] certain mistrust of what my body was doing. So that was a really difficult place, especially after I feel like I had been through some really transformative experiences in those months. I was tired from going through the first loss. **Lexi**

When grief intersected with issues of silence and failure, isolation added itself to the experience. Lisa and Jenn both described how loneliness affected them:

So it [was] just really, really hard. And it just felt like really desperate; I felt really desperate and I felt really alone. **Lisa**

The biggest thing that would help is if people talk about it. One thing that was really hard for me with the late one was reaching the due date and not being pregnant again or anything like that. The one that I lost late, I was due right before Thanksgiving. It was the day before Thanksgiving. So when that date came around…and what made it worse is that I started my period on the date that she would have been due…that was hard. Because it was so late it felt a lot more real to me because I got to see the baby but…it didn't seem as real to other people as it did to me. It would have made me feel better if I had known that other people recognized that date. And that would have been a due date and I would have had a baby at that time. And my husband hadn't been that helpful to me because I felt so alone. I think he knew that it was the due date but he didn't say anything about it. And…so I felt really kind of alone at that point because no one acknowledged it, which I can understand because I don't know how people would have felt about bringing it up. And it wasn't a big date that I could remember anyways but it would have been nice and helpful for me if someone would have acknowledged it and acknowledged what I was going through at that time. **Jenn**

One problem with involuntary pregnancy loss is that just because you experienced one does not mean that the world will momentarily stop having babies. Susan and Shannon both described the experience of running into such a cold fact after their loss:

*Yeah it's…kind a full circle thing because now I feel like…I have it every once in a while. It still comes you know…sometimes I'll see something like a couple coming out of their ultrasound. And they're so happy looking at their picture like 'look at that little flutter'. And it hurts but then you are okay you know…it's just like a little sadness that you have to live with…***Susan**

Sometimes I feel like tattooing it on my forehead to shove it in people's faces. I no longer smile when I see a pregnant woman. It makes me sad and angry. I have a hard time feeling happy for people I know who are expecting or have recently given birth. I feel a lot of jealousy instead. **Shannon**

Listening to and quantifying grief are similar in that both fail to comprehensively understand it. Although scientific literature can offer visual evidence of the impacts of miscarriage on a woman's life, to just approach the topic within the realm of objectivity leaves out the rest of the story. Quantifying sadness homogenizes the experience and takes away the individual value. Simply put, "...it would be difficult and unfair to define, catalog, or quantify the emotional impact of pregnancy loss in any standardizing way" (Berman, 2001:93). In addition, attempts to comprehend another's pain through listening runs the risk of projecting one's own perceptions and contexts into the situation. Assuming that one can fully understand another's experience only results in a destruction of communication. Trying to fully comprehend grief is no different than trying to build the tower of Babel.

The best that one can do in order to grasp basic concepts of such pain is to combine the personal experiences of women with the quantification of what grief is supposed to be. For example, in her analysis of the phases those women go through during involuntary pregnancy loss, Wright (2010) found that many women experience an initial reaction of numbness. This is similar to Susan's description of how initially she had more of a delayed reaction.

Another good study to compare with these women's stories is *"Guilt and emptiness: women's experiences with miscarriage"* by Adolfsson et al. (2004), which aimed to "identify and describe the women's experiences of miscarriage..." (545) in an effort to categorize common emotions. One main theme identified was emptiness, or the state of being in which a woman is reacting to her loss and exhibits depressive symptoms. Although ll of the women interviewed grieved after their loss in different ways, several common themes and their subsequent consequences surfaced. For example, a strong feeling of abandonment resulted from interactions between the woman and her support structures (Adolfsson et al., 2004). This is similar to Lisa's experience. Her negative interactions from family as well as in the hospital in Puerto Rico (her support structures) were a factor in why she *"felt really desperate* and...really alone". In contrast, Jenn had a solid support structure. Her feeling of isolation did not come from lack of support, but from the lack of acknowledgement of her due date. Abandonment in this case was not a matter of support levels; it was one of visual validation.

Adolfsson et al. (2004) also identified perceptions that the community discounted the intensity of women's sadness if they already had children. This was similarly true for Jenni, who described the unusual pattern that grief takes. When something triggers a resurgence of grief after the acceptable period of mourning has passed, others discount it with comments of "you've come to have two more children".

Verbalized abandonment occurred when family members and friends mourned the loss faster than the woman did and expected her to stop grieving at a certain point (Adolfsson et al., 2004). This conflict is similar to what Jenni described. In terms of limitations on mourning, she felt that "There's a stigma in...grief. In grieving for too long". However, unlike the study findings, she provided an explanation for why this conflict occurs:

> When you've lost a child, I'm not sure that the grief process ever fully ends because the love for the child and the sadness that you feel that the child isn't here is so intertwined. It is very difficult to ask a mother to give up grieving because it feels like you're asking them to give up the loving...which isn't going to happen. **Jenni**

The idea that grief is a pattern that occurs in linear shifts after a miscarriage has also had its share of scientific analysis. Swanson et al. (2007) interviewed women at one, six, sixteen, and fifty-two weeks post-pregnancy loss in an effort to understand the gradual trend of a woman's grief after a pregnancy loss. With the exception of a few women in the study, the researchers determined the pattern of grief to be an overall shift from active grieving to general acceptance.

Although this study had a strong design, was statistically significant and acknowledged that some women do not follow this trend, the quantification alone of a "grief pattern" standardizes mourning guidelines for miscarriage. In explaining her surprise at the grieving process Jenni told me:

I didn't have any sense of what the grieving process is like. And I will just say that it is nothing like the five stages in my personal [opinion]. **Jenni**

As someone who has gone through a different kind of grieving process in the past two years, I made a wave motion with my hand and asked her if that is how it felt. She laughed and said, *"Actually it's more like this".* She then drew a downward spiral in the air. Perhaps it is simply interpretation of how hands tell no lies, but I am fairly sure that a gradual linear trend of grief is quite different than one that looks very much like a spiral downward.

Before and After

After women had described their experience with pregnancy loss I asked them how it had changed their lives. Several felt that they were "profoundly affected" by their losses, to the point of it being a changing moment in their lives:

There is just a difference in women who have had this kind of pregnancy loss. And it's interesting and I'm interested to know why you're focusing more on [involuntary pregnancy loss] before twenty weeks. It's kind of like before and after. Like you have this life before and then you have the life after. I think it's true for anyone with pregnancy loss, no matter when it was…it's forever changing you in a way you can't really experience. It's actually very similar to the loss of a mother. I lost my mother so I can say that it was very similar like 'this is how it was, and [now] this is how it is.' And you walk around in this daze wondering why people are asking you what time it is. Or you know, 'why did that person cut me off in traffic cause don't they know my daughter died'. **Lisa**

[It affected me] really in every way. I think…I talked about this with other friends that have been through this. On the pregnancy loss track, like this is pretty new. Even though I'm almost at the two-year mark. So…I don't feel very connected to the person who I was before this happened. And I understand that over time those experiences sort of get integrated but part of what my experience was like was that it was…it was genuine trauma. I was diagnosed with posttraumatic anxiety afterwards. I became dissociative; I

had social anxiety. It kind of fundamentally rocked the way that I… perceived my own safety and the safety of my family in the world. And how I perceived authority figures and medical people…it's very very far reaching, that sense of…having the rug pulled out from under you. So in that sense it's really…touched everything in my life. And not necessarily for the better. **Jenni**

I would say that I have been utterly and profoundly affected by my losses…in ways that I don't know that I can yet anticipate how they will affect me as a parent. And as a partner. And maybe as a person. **Lexi**

It's changed everything about me, how I feel about my life and my family, how my career has changed, and my relationship with my husband. Unfortunately, [with my] pregnancy loss, there isn't a single puzzle piece I could lift out of my life. Or somehow go back in time four years to when I was happy and thought everything in my life was going perfectly. I used to pride myself on my health. While my husband has type 1 diabetes and everyone in his family has had some sort of cancer or ailment. I don't even wear glasses. Now I think about how if it weren't for my fertility issues I would still think I had above average health. It's hard to feel that way when your uterus kills babies. **Shannon**

I understand pain that other people go through more. I understand what loss is, so I feel like I have an understanding of some of the darkness that there is in life. More than I did before. **Kirsten**

I received varied answers from the women when I asked how pregnancy loss had affected their lives. For some it marked the fundamental shift not only in them, but also in how they interacted with the world. Lisa will always see her existence through the lens of before and after. Lexi was also radically changed, though she is still waiting to see just how the loss will affect her perceptions of the roles she fills in her life. For some women, the loss affected them in significantly traumatic ways. Jenni experienced post-traumatic and social anxiety, a sense of dissociation, and a loss of confidence in the safety of those around her. For Shannon, her losses negatively impacted her physical health, her mental health, and her overall happiness.

In general, all of the women seemed to gain a sort of melancholy omniscience. I remember being struck by Kirsten's comment that she had gained *"an understanding of some of the darkness that there is in this world"*. I think Lisa found the same sight when her concepts of what was important in life shifted. Lexi found it in the knowledge that the roles in her life had fundamentally changed and would continue to. Jenn found it in her disconnection to her former self. Shannon sees it when she looks back and recognizes that she used to be happy.

I feel that knowledge of certain types of grief can be a fickle thing. Having such an experience can allow one to perceive moments and situations that would be impossible to recognize otherwise. However, this knowledge may also cause a sense of nostalgic hindsight. After a certain level of grief, one may have trouble approaching certain situations in the same way as before. Such experiences can also characterize once happy moments as incidents leading up to loss. For example, a woman who was elated to be pregnant and experienced an involuntary pregnancy loss may no longer look back on those moments as joyful. Grief is fickle because it does necessarily stay within the boundaries of its own experience.

Stigma

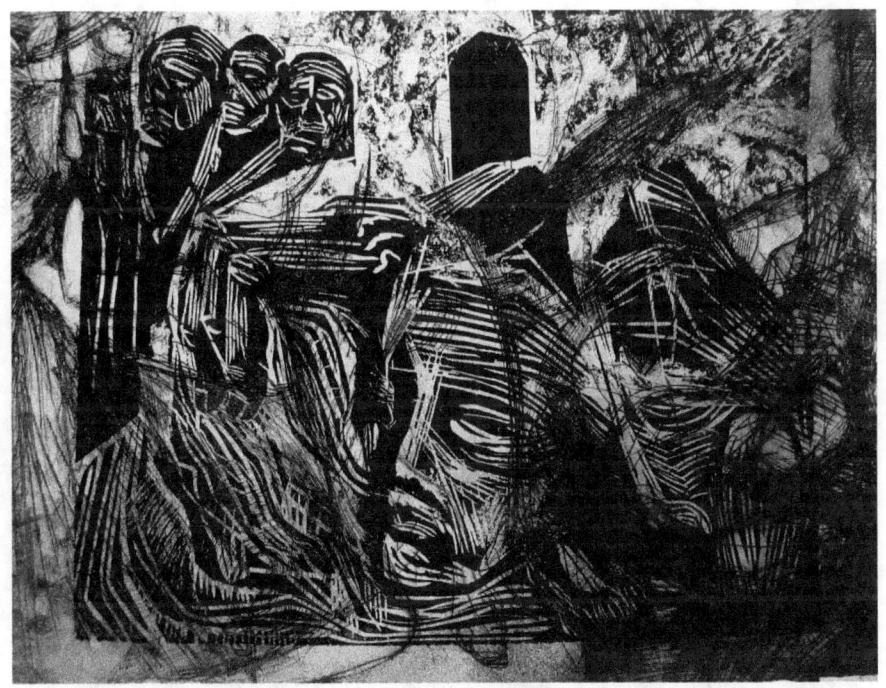

Stigma was the main theme I expected to find in my interviews. What I unearthed was quite different than what I had imagined. I had been accurate in guessing that a lot of women dealt with the concept of failure. What I misjudged was how much shame women felt and why they felt it. From what I could tell, women within the pregnancy loss community do talk about their experiences. The problem is, they only feel comfortable talking about them with each other. Shame starts to exist the farther you get away from a community that understands the experience.

Under the context of stigma I found several things. Within the community I found a commentary on how much the idea of failure plays into personal experience. The process and decision to tell others about the loss brought up several aspects of this. I found the connection between reactions to opening up about losses and silence. Finally, I discovered how the women perceived silence's effect on them and how they wanted to remove the stigma around their experience.

Failure to produce

A lot of the women I interviewed mentioned the concern that their bodies would not ever be able to successfully carry a child:

> Well we were kind of wondering, you know. It seemed to be a pretty sure thing (laughs) a couple things...you know, is this is the way it was going to be, are we not going to be able to conceive a child? To hold it full term or not, you know? **Cindy**

> I think especially after I had the second one right close after the first one, I kind of felt...felt like there was something wrong maybe. That I wasn't able to have kids. **Amber**

> ...I felt like I should have been able to carry that baby. **Jennifer**

> And...I you know I just was always kind of nervous that it was going to happen again. I mean you really feel very very fragile and you feel, that the baby is really vulnerable. I guess that one, I was a lot more worried about the possibility that things would not work out. And then when I did...I was really, the most devastated...with the second miscarriage because I really thought that maybe this was just going to keep happening and that we were never going to have kids. **Amy**

In addition to explaining how not being able to carry a pregnancy to term created a sense of personal failure, Jenni also described the anxiety of being seen by the world only as someone who miscarried:

> Yeah...I mean there's a huge sense that my body totally failed. Partly because of how she died, you know my body basically...as far as we know there wasn't anything wrong with her, it's just my body couldn't carry the pregnancy. So

that was kind of difficult…I still quite haven't made my peace with that aspect of it. And then there's the not wanting to be that girl. I've heard other moms talk about this too, it's like 'wow for the rest of my life I am always going to be seen as the girl whose baby died or the girl who had this terrible miscarriage or the girl whose baby died and then she couldn't get pregnant again. And there's I think a lot of social…images of the sort of Victorian woman who is infertile or who has a stillborn baby and goes insane. You know, and so that kind of…resonates in a way because you really do feel like you've gone insane and then you think like "wow I'm the girl who went crazy because her baby died." **Jenni**

Susan and Kirsten both described running into the stigma associated with being married and not having children:

I think I did for a while; feel stigmatized. I remember someone finding out that I'd been married for four years and didn't have a child. She looked at me and said 'well do you want children?" As if I'd done something. And I was really irritated; it was none of her business. You have no idea what people have to deal with, how could you even ask such a question? …But of course I was more defensive about it in my head than I was actually to her. But for a while I kind of felt like 'what did I do, what…what's wrong with me and how come I can't pull this off when most people can?' A lot of people I knew had babies by accident. It didn't seem fair. So I, I wonder if the choices I had made had led up to this and I did feel a bit of shame towards it. **Kirsten**

You get that message like [the one] I got from my doctor's office. The only person who would talk about it…because I knew at forty-three I was aware of [the risks] but…I think there's…only when you're not faced with that pressure 'you're supposed to have kids' and you don't, people wonder like… are you selfish or is there something wrong biologically? They feel sorry for you. **Susan**

Cindy, Amber, and Amy all mentioned their past anxieties over whether or not they would ever be able to have children. The phrasing of their fears, however, placed the fault of the miscarriage on the failure of the body. For many, pregnancy was a state and it was up to their body "*to hold it full term*". Amber felt that something was "*wrong*", and Jenni felt that her "*body totally failed*". Embedded in these expressions is the social expectation that these women *"should have been able to carry that baby"*. Such language implies that women control their body and should feel guilty for failing.

Failing to have a successful childbirth is seen as a horrible reflection on the woman because it culturally negates her role as one. As was mentioned in the explanation of success, an American woman has historically been defined by her ability to reproduce (Weitz, 2003). Also previously mentioned in the discussion on power was the notion that pregnancy is considered a rite of passage in which the woman assumes her role in society as a valid individual. Rites and rituals are significant because they instill symbolic meaning in those that participate and those that observe. A disruption in this communication still relays a very symbolic message, that of failure. Whereas normal information that is relayed can be approached in a systematic way, symbols are "...*felt* in its totality through the body and the emotions..." (Davis-Floyd, 2003:9). And totality is extremely difficult to systematically explain and diffuse. Taboos of this sort are therefore much harder to remove from society's general assumption because they are not simply analytic.

A rite of passage is as important for the individual as it is for the community in which it is performed. Davis-Floyd (2003) cites Munn in explaining: "rituals work to align the belief system of the individual with that of the social group conducting the ritual" (10). As a result, some women, such as Jenni, worry that their lack of success means that they will always be known by their failure:

> *...You really do feel like you've gone insane and then you think like "wow I'm the girl who went crazy because her baby died."* **Jenni**

Conflicts within women's health movements may also play a role in enforcing identification of the self as a failure. Autonomy is an incredible tool, but it can be a double-edged sword. Several of the women I interviewed as well as myself live in an area where alternative and natural methods to pregnancy birth are prevalent. As wonderful as the natural birth movement is, the expectations and assumptions placed on the act and outcome of pregnancy and birth are as rigid as the more medically centered model. In asserting that birth is always natural and that the woman is in complete control of the body, the movement places the pregnancy loss experience in a conundrum: "Either women accept responsibility for the pregnancy loss and blame themselves for the death of the 'baby', or they must admit that the loss was a bodily event over which they had no control" (Layne, 2003:19).

Failure is, ironically, the fertile seed of shame. In addition to emptiness and guilt, blame was a main theme identified in the study by Adolfsson et al. (2004). The combination of these results...resulted in the conclusion that "...women do not only feel the loss of an early pregnancy but also the loss of a baby, an expected child, their motherhood, their self-esteem, and their ability to be able to reproduce themselves" (556).

In general, the women attempted to identify which of their actions caused the loss (such as smoking, drinking, etc.), which resulted in a strong sense of self-blame. Kirsten experienced a similar type of self-blame in wondering, *"if the choices I had made had led up to this"*. The Adolfsson (2004) study subjects also placed a significant level of personal and community expectation on the ability to have children. This social pressure is very similar to the one felt by Susan, who faced the taboo of being married without children. Talk about a damned if you do, damned if you don't scenario. As she has been married for a culturally significant amount of time and has still not had children, she is seen as selfish. However, if she were to explain that she is unable to have them, she would be seen as a failure as a woman, as a wife, and as a member of her community. Whatever the reason for the lack of children, society deems it an individual's fault.

Letting others in on what happened

Having grasped a basic understanding of the implications of involuntary pregnancy loss in terms of failure and stigma, I asked the women if they had told others about their experience. Jenni told as many people as possible as soon as she could:

I just, I felt this sudden overwhelming need for everyone to know as soon as possible...I didn't want, a month later, to be in some situation where someone said 'weren't you pregnant?' or 'did you have the baby?' It was such this huge thing, like the next day that was heavy on my mind so I just kind of activated my social network and was like 'please tell anyone who knows me that this is what happened.' Which isn't really the way that it's...you know, I was like 'I have to break silence about this because otherwise I will get screwed at some point and have a nervous breakdown in public so I just want everyone to know'. (laughs) **Jenni**

Kirsten talked to women who had already gone through the experience:

Well the first one, I talked to other people that had [experienced] a loss. I remember a lot of the nurses told me their experiences while I was in the hospital. It was just a short time but I felt comfortable about that. And talking to my mother about her experience helped. And I had another friend too who had been pregnant and then lost hers. We talked about that and then I had another friend who, we were pregnant at the same time. And she continued on to have a baby. And she brought me dinner and I just felt like these were...reaching out to other women was mainly the way that I dealt with it. That and sleeping. **Kirsten**

Shannon preferred to hold off telling others unless she had gotten to know them:

I'm not sure how my interactions with the community have changed or been impacted. I don't blurt out my losses when I first meet someone, but after getting to know someone I will tell them about it. Especially if they are the type to go on and on about their children or pregnancy experiences. I get the impression that they think I have no clue about any of these things since I already told them I don't have kids. That doesn't mean I haven't been pregnant...I cried a lot, I still do sometimes if I'm talking about it with someone new. It's easier to talk about my losses without crying with people I've already broken the news to. **Shannon**

In general, open conversation about involuntary pregnancy loss received very shocked and uncomfortable responses. Through the explanation of a running joke she and her husband had after her loss, Lexi summed up the general consensus on openly talking about involuntary pregnancy loss:

Yeah I mean it's funny because people send out their

Christmas cards every year, like 'our family year in review'. My husband and I keep joking like wow I could just write a super somber piece of recounting the year that just...I mean it was such a messy messy...year and I, I think 'oh God nobody would read this'...(laughs) 'nobody would read this. They would throw me away and then they would remove me from their card list for the rest of their lives'. **Lexi**

As a result of the reactions to their initial news both Jenni and Shannon changed how they brought up the subject, if they did at all:

I found that, with my group of friends in particular, that people just get really uncomfortable if I bring it up. I become extremely hesitant to bring it up and if I do...I carefully contextualize it, which I'm able to do now but within the first year I couldn't...be careful with them. So I ended up really not talking about it very much. I mostly talked about it with my family or with my new friends on the internet, which were really like my big support system. **Jenni**

I also don't bother to tell my in-laws when I'm pregnant since they wouldn't be sympathetic if I had another loss. **Shannon**

Scientific literature on communication about pregnancy loss places a major emphasis on its importance for the psyche of the woman. For example, Berman (2001) found that "The context in which the loss is perceived by the mother and her ability to freely communicate how she is feeling may contribute to her long term adjustment" (91).

What I am learning quickly throughout this project is how important the difference between telling someone about the occurrence and actually talking about the experience is. One could look at these narratives and assume that women were open about their loss. However, for several the goal was to alert others as soon as possible so that they wouldn't have to explain any further. For example, Jenni tried to let "*everyone know as soon as possible*" so that she would not be caught off guard if someone asked her about her pregnancy. Lisa sent out an email so that everyone knew not to approach her. Both women told others, but they did not talk to them about it or even try to explain the experience.

The literature seems to be universal in assuming that all silence in negative (St. John et al., 2006). However, when you compare this idea to the women's narratives, Initial silence may actually be beneficial. In order to open up about what happened, women need to first go through their own experience. The silence that exists immediately after the news has been broken may allow the woman time to ground herself. The conflict occurs when the woman are finally ready to talk about their loss, but no one is ready to listen. This is evident in Lexi's assumption that incorporating the news of her loss within the rest of her life experiences that year would completely ostracize her. Society is all right with being told the initial news, but only if it is described as a separate event from the rest of the woman and the community's lives.

We don't talk about that, but we should

Overall, the general message that most of the interviewed women received was that miscarriage was a failure on their part and that the rest of the world did not want to talk openly about it:

> ...As a pregnancy editor I know all the statistics. One in four women lose a baby. Except I don't know of that one person who talks about it among my four friends. So I think that is really difficult to me to sort of experience...it felt very isolating at the time. **Lexi**

However, all of the women felt that just because it was the norm did not mean that this kind of cultural expectation was in any way acceptable:

> I would be very aware...it's something that people don't openly talk about...I know a friend, a nurse at the doctors office, being like 'don't tell too many people because if it doesn't work out...you won't want to talk about it, you might not want to talk about it'. You just get that message of it's not okay...and I think that's why. It's something that you go through. You don't have to tell every person in the world but you should be able to talk about it...I just wish that I could have been more open. That I had been allowed to be...I was suffering and I didn't feel like I could tell anybody, you know? **Susan**

> After my second loss I began sort of...searching for people who would let me talk about something that I just felt needed

to be discussed really bad. And I have found that… I began blogging for Parenting.com at the very beginning of my second trimester. And I have found people who I never in a million years would have expected. I mean, bosses I had fifteen years ago, you know? People who I worked with in high school have come out of the woodwork saying 'I also had two pregnancy losses and I now have four kids'. And I'm so glad to be talking about it. I don't think I'm affecting change, but I do think I'm changing the way that I feel about how…people will respond to other people's openness about hard stuff…We have such a really crafty way of dealing with, discussing loss in this country…pregnancy loss and death, and you know, and older people death, and all sorts of loss. But I think especially around [pregnancy loss], we've got ways to go. And I am hopeful that people will make that change…I can see that there are, you know…thriving online communities of people who are discussing loss. But hardly any of those people are surrounded by that kind of support in their real life…I, I am actually more ashamed of not being…I would say the only shame I felt is not being more forthcoming both times with the greater community around me because I think that if we don't talk about miscarriage were not going to talk about miscarriage. **Lexi**

You're never completely open about it. It happens so often to so many people, it feels like you should talk about it…I think when it happens and you…understand that this is something that happens quite frequently, you can really start to talk about it. **Amy**

It comes as no surprise that involuntary pregnancy loss is not talked about in the general culture. Even the pregnancy resources skip over it. Some of the women I talked to described what was available to them when they needed information:

I read a couple books but it was mainly about the pregnancy…I really read the parts about experiencing loss and…It kind of seems like in the pregnancy books [the] subject is really taboo. They don't really want to talk about it too much because most everyone who is…who is reading it is filled with all this joy. **Malissa**

It's not something you even want to think about when you're pregnant for the first time. You skip over those parts in your pregnancy books. **Shannon**

I have felt that there are so few fluent resources out there. And I think that women who are in the process of miscarrying are hungry for stories. Because there are so few...you know it's hard. I've also felt like a tool of the system before because as a parenting editor I've worked for most of the major parenting and pregnancy websites and those are created to foster community around pregnancy. And the moment that you lose a baby, you suddenly have no resources at all to give you [information on] what comes next. And it is a shame. It is a product of marketing. And a business issue that is greater than any one company is going to tackle. It's like 'who is going to sponsor the website about dead babies'? Not the formula companies. So it is a big issue and it's something that people need to address...I want there to be more people talking about this. **Lexi**

The warning Susan received about telling too many people about her early pregnancy suggests that it is not the woman staying silent that creates silence. It is that society does not want to (and does not feel like it is allowed to) listen. The suggestion that one does not tell others they are pregnant until they are reasonably far along is a common one. Why though? Does this precaution exist to shield the community from having to deal with the grief if there is a loss during the early parts of the pregnancy? As the facilitator of the SHARE group explained, a taboo on the visibility of early pregnancy places a woman in a position of silence. You cannot explain to your family and friends that you are going through a pregnancy loss if you never told them you were pregnant in the first place.

The opposite aspect of this is also true. Women often experience guilt when they have told others about their pregnancy and then have a pregnancy loss. In her memoir, A Perfect Replica of a Figment of My Imagination, McCracken (2008) describes her immediate thought at the moment of loss that is all too common: "I knew, I knew, that this was all my fault. My essential reaction was grief, but somehow the words that floated to the surface of my brain were: people are going to be mad at me" (154-5).

The penalty of guilt for acknowledging loss is a reflection on cultural attitudes of grief. Kluger-Bell (1998) found that "Often, by minimizing the impact of significant losses, pathologizing those whose reactions are intense, and applauding those who seem relatively unaffected by tragic events, we encourage the inhibition of our own grief" (22). Still, sentiments such as McCracken's bring up several questions about the cultural influences on the experience of silence. How is society constructed in a way that women feel obligated to their community to have a healthy pregnancy? What does this say about pregnancy as a responsibility and a signifier of womanhood? And finally, what does this say about society's perception of women in general?

Loss is definitely not an easy topic for the speaker. For the listener, it is difficult because it brings sadness for the other and illuminates possible flaws within the self. "It is uncomfortable to witness the suffering of others: it makes us aware of how powerless we are to control so many aspects of our lives" (Kluger-Bell 1998:15). Pregnancy loss can be a sad, if not a sometimes-devastating thing and our culture often places great authority in knowledge of pain and the power of intention. This shifts the pregnancy loss experience from a significant event in one's life to that of a forewarning. After her loss, McCracken (2008) found that

I am that thing worse than a cautionary tale: I am a horror story, an example of something terrible going wrong when you least expect it, and for no good reason, a story to be kept from pregnant women, a story so grim and lesson less it's better not to think about at all. (43)

Certain deaths, like that of a mother and father, are for the most part inevitable. Condolence for such loss is simply preparation for your own grief when things take a turn for the worse, and we must acknowledge that which is a mandatory life event. In contrast, pregnancy loss is not inevitable-if you try to avoid talking to those it has happened to and your card is not the one in four, it is possible to go an entire lifespan without running into such sentiments. As Linda Layne (2003) explains with a quote from Aries, culturally we live with an "interdiction of death" (66): "There is a modern 'need for happiness-the moral duty and the social obligation to contribute to the collective happiness by avoiding any cause for sadness of boredom..." (66). Of course no one talks about it. In the utilitarian frame of things, sadness is a grievance towards greater society. And the best way to discourage such behavior is to stigmatize it.

Distance

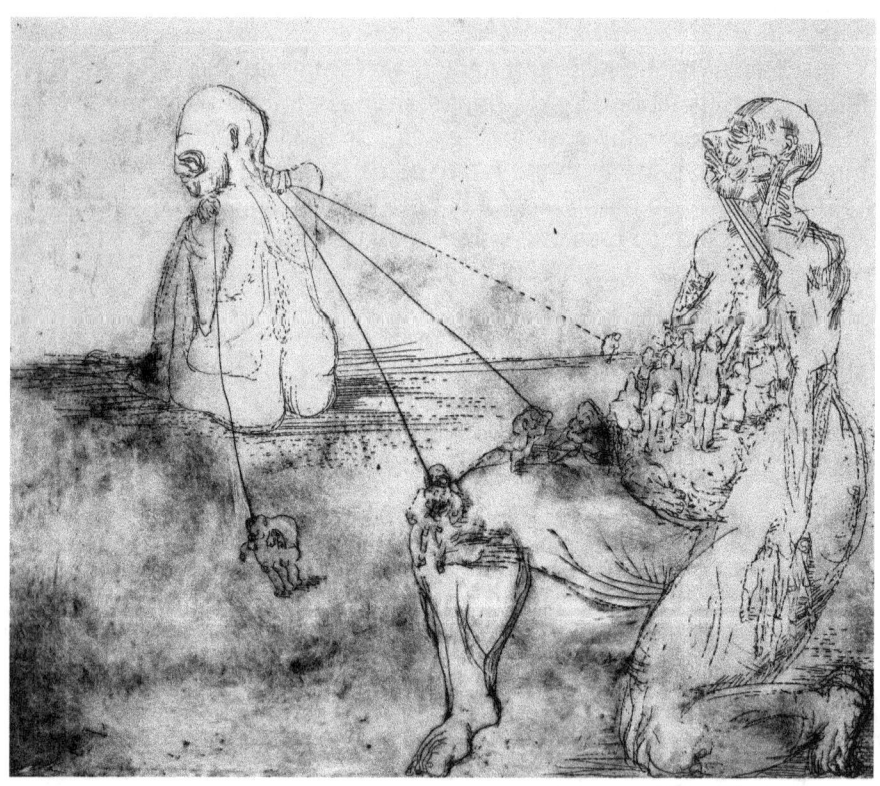

    In the midst of going through my research and transcripts to
sketch out main themes, I kept finding myself separating ideas in
terms of us vs. them. Distance is a unique concept in that it exists in
every topic I have come across. The results from my interviews
have made me wonder how one's experience and understanding of
miscarriage can create a divide between oneself and others. How
you perceive your own power and the power around you comes
under a completely different context. Pain has a new meaning that
few others, if anyone, can fully understand. Stigma, both in how you

perceive it and what it means at its very core, is a completely different beast.

Distance can sometimes involve differences between parties that are most evident within conflict. The women I talked to discovered them in their interactions with their healthcare providers, family, partners and community. The circle of shared experience that they now belong to was sometimes embedded with the idea that you can only understand once you have already experienced the event. In being defined by difference and contrast, I found that the women also shifted their experience of what was similar. Other women with parallel experiences suddenly came out of the woodwork. Distance is a focus on how an event within you can fundamentally transform the proximity of the life outside of you.

US vs. Them: Healthcare

If no one around you can relate to your experience, how would you even know there was a miscarriage community? The answer is evident in the experiences with the healthcare system (that many of the women had). There seemed to be a major contrast between providers who did not know what to do and other healthcare workers whose experience helped to somewhat alleviate the situation:

I had great interactions with healthcare other than one…one person since you asked the question. There was one doctor at my OB who when I first had the blood clot said to me 'well you have a 50-50 chance of losing the pregnancy' and it upset me so much that I no longer would make appointments when she would be there. I would schedule my appointments when she didn't work. There was sort of like a group, you would just go in with whomever. And then lo and behold when I delivered the baby…my doctor induced labor and I was in labor for eighteen hours. So he was there for twelve of them. But then he had to go and lo and behold she was the person on call so she was the one who delivered the baby. Which really sucked. And then she was just like really weird about it, she didn't…she I mean she's been through pregnancy loss but [she's] not familiar with delivering a baby at nineteen weeks. So when I delivered the baby and she died in childbirth she tried to put the baby in a *stainless steel bowl to present to me. And that was really upsetting...it was just a weird situation and the nurse kind of handled the situation. But in my subsequent pregnancy I refused to see her. I just would not see her and any time anybody asked what the issue was I would just blurt out everything that she had done and...I don't know I mean I'm sure it got back to her but... **Lisa***

*I got sick and they didn't know what was wrong...and it's just really a weird thing because I remember having the ultrasound and the ultrasound tech...I know there's something wrong because I can tell by the look on her face and all of a sudden she stopped talking. And she was acting really weird and then she left the room. And I was like 'okay so now I have to wait for the doctor to decide to come in'. So then...it took a really long time, you know. Something that really shouldn't happen, you shouldn't...she should have been a little less awkward about it. **Cindy***

*The doctor gets me on the phone...they called me into the doctor's office. And he starts hollering at me: 'you weren't supposed to get pregnant! I told you not to get pregnant!' and all this stuff, you know? Anyways...it was just like all that stuff was not a good experience; it was not fun. **Cindy***

*With my first two miscarriages the healthcare was horrible. The doctor I had, she had a horrible bedside manner; she wasn't sympathetic at all. She wasn't comforting at all. She was pretty cold and...and so I changed doctors immediately and...he was amazing. He was absolutely amazing. And so...the first two [miscarriages] were horrible, and the second two I went to another doctor. It was the same hospital but a new doctor and it was a lot better. The nurses were great, they gave me book; they sent home a little figurine. **Jenn***

*It would be nice if they would just tell you rather than jerk you around and send you back to your doctor's office to wait in the waiting room full of happy pregnant women while you cry about your latest dead baby...the ultrasound tech actually left the room to find a doctor to discuss "my case" with me and left the vaginal probe for the ultrasound inside me while she was gone. **Shannon***

93

In addition to feeling like their healthcare providers were insensitive, Lisa and Jenni had experiences where it seemed as if no one cared about the situation. Both women felt completely exasperated by the nonchalance of others:

I think that... [With] most of my friends it's hard to say. Some of my friends were really very just there and very supportive. They would call me every day when I was in the hospital. Other friends...didn't call. Or said they would call...supposedly there was a treatment for a torn amniotic sac, like 'you can repair it and there's this doctor in Colorado' and all this stuff. And this friend was like 'oh I'll look into it' and she just never did. And she just never called me back. So I'm in the hospital desperate to save this bab- this pregnancy and she just, you know, I was just so uncomfortable...She just didn't call back or...didn't have the same...sense of urgency that I felt. So that was very disconcerting and disappointing. **Lisa**

And you know it's the worst of it where you start bleeding at midnight and you have to go in to the emergency room at one AM and it's like the worst time to be in the emergency room. So all kinds of crazy stuff happened. Like I saw seven doctors in five hours and then they couldn't be in one mind. I got into a turf war between the doctor who thought my cervix was funneling and the doctor who [didn't]...that doctor was like a young jock trying to move up in the ranks. And then...I got abandoned in one of the rooms on the ward. They thought that radiology was coming for me, but radiology didn't know where I was. I had an IV in my arm and my call bell was unplugged. And I actually ended up like driving my IV thing, like down into the hallway into the lobby because I had to pee. So there were just a lot of aspects of like...'I'm trying to keep a baby alive here'. And nobody is kind of getting on board with the urgency of that project. **Jenni**

Miscommunication and conflict between women who are experiencing involuntary pregnancy loss and their healthcare providers is a perfect example of what happens when two groups without each other's knowledge and experience must interact. Surveys of patient satisfaction following miscarriage have indicated a high percentage of anger and dissatisfaction with the medical care received. The main complaints centered on physician insensitivity and lack of opportunity to discuss the personal significance of the loss (Brier, 1999). When women such as Lisa are told that they have a chance of losing the pregnancy without any other information, major conflict occurs. Additionally, when providers are not educated about sensitivity and what an involuntary pregnancy loss can mean to a woman, occurrences such as putting *"the baby in a stainless steel bowl to present to me"* will be much more common.

The medical community is still trying to determine if giving out all of the scientific information about what is going on is beneficial. *"Distress after miscarriage: relation to the knowledge of the cause of pregnancy loss and coping style"* by Nikčević et al. (2003) analyzed how a woman's awareness about what caused her pregnancy loss affected both her reaction to the event and her coping mechanisms. The study hypothesized that some women (monitors) want to know as much information as possible but others (blunters) do not want to know the details. If these concepts were correct, giving women detailed information about the physiological reasons for their pregnancy loss would result in an increase in distress (compared to normal reactions) for a blunter and a decrease in distress for a monitor. Contrary to the hypothesis, they found that an informational follow-up session after a pregnancy loss that includes information and support significantly decreased anxiety and helped coping mechanisms overall (Nikčević et al., 2003).

In another study, Nikčević (2003) found that women who used a follow up service reported faster levels of emotional recovery compared to women who did not. In trying to determine if medical or psychological counseling was independently responsible for positive outcomes, they found that psychological counseling and both types used together are beneficial but medical counseling alone may increase distress.

Information for the families and women who experience pregnancy loss is extremely important, as it allows them to better understand what is occurring in the situation and leaves them with more of a feeling of control. This is especially true in interactions with the healthcare system, where the woman is already ceding control by allowing others to alter her body. As is also evident by the women's stories, medical information or general information alone makes the situation worse. It was the providers that told the women what was happening, were aware of the sensitivity and emotional aspects of the situation, and who treated their patients with respect that helped to create a good healthcare experience.

Us vs. Them: male partners and family

One area I found interesting was how the relationship between the women and the male members of their family shifted as a result of the loss. I wanted to know if the lack of even a possibility of loss created a difference in interactions between these members and family who could become pregnant. A review of the literature by Klier et al. (2002) concluded "miscarriage may have a greater impact on the woman because she carries the pregnancy, biologically as well as symbolically" (141). I wanted to see if my results reflected this idea:

My dad really doesn't get it. Like...he views it as...something...a medical problem that happened to me. And [he] is concerned for my safety and wellbeing, which is very nice. He's not mean about it but he's just...there's a disconnect for him in terms of what I'm experiencing. Like he sent me a get well soon card after instead of a sympathy card. It's like there's a little bit of a lack in understanding. **Jenni**

I think...[my husband] was upset too. And I think initially...he had to support me and it was...this thing with me like checking in with me, but [he was] not really involved with it. Like I said it was afterwards that...for some reason it took a few weeks for me to actually...I think that's when it really started to hit me... I think he just didn't know how to [deal with that] basically...so we had to work through that...and then it took us so long because we had gone through so much that we just kind of needed a break from everything. To decide what to do. **Susan**

My dad was just like 'well now that that's over you know you can...you can go on a diet and lose weight'. He wasn't...he didn't understand at all and it...caused a really uncomfortable rift between my father and I...my husband was really, I can see he really just rose to the occasion when I was in the hospital... **Lisa**

I would say that my husband and I had what I would

consider to be a typical bout of miscommunication. And it was a really difficult time. But in general I would say things were really messy for about three months after my first pregnancy. And then it was really difficult. I think that it was an experience that he felt like he couldn't have a lot of physical connection to. And so some of the emotional reaction that I was having he just couldn't latch onto...we did seek really great therapy. I'm a huge believer in therapy. And ...that was relationship changing. I mean just a real game changer for the two of us. **Lexi**

They were parallel but they were very different; the ways that we grieved. And it...did create problems for a little while. I mean we had the initial insanity of...being very newly married and we had actually only known each other for eight months before we got married so we were in a brand new relationship...although interestingly before this happened we had already been through the death of his brother-in-law, a cancer scare for his father and he had hernia surgery (laughs) so that was all within the first three months of our marriage. So we weren't completely untested but we were fairly untested when this happened. And he did the guy thing of like 'I must work all the time now'. And he was just...completely in work mode and he just went into the zone of like 'I have to work I have to work even harder...I have to keep the roof over our heads and pay the bills and keep life from completely imploding'. And I was home alone most of the day and was just completely devastated and [it] was made worse by his absence. But there was a period of time where we were really like this (hands far apart) but we kind of eased back together. **Jenni**

There seems to be dissimilarity between how male members of a woman's family experience pregnancy. For Lexi's partner, the experience was one that "*he felt like he couldn't have a lot of physical connection to*". The fact that he had not and could never physically know what it felt like to be or to connect to a pregnancy was a significant factor in "*things being really messy for about three months after*" Lexi's pregnancy.

In contrast, the pregnancy loss had a huge physical effect on Jenni's partner. This experience is consistent with much of the literature about how the male partner is affected. In "*A grief ignored:*

narratives of pregnancy loss from a male perspective", McCreight (2004) conducted extensive and long-term (once a month for three years) interviews with men who attended a pregnancy loss support group. Midwives and nurses were also interviewed to get a perception of the men from a (assumed) female provider's perspective. Although the time since the miscarriage (or stillbirth) had occurred ranged from two months to twenty years, the interview was the first time that many of these men had been directly asked about their own personal experience in the situation.

All of the men vocalized having identified with the fetus as their baby, partially blamed themselves for the loss of the pregnancy (for situations such as not noticing warning signs or not listening to their partners closely enough) and were not sure if they could consider themselves legitimate fathers if they did not have any living children. They also felt that they had lost the chance of fatherhood as a conceivable possibility, were affected if they were not socially recognized as the legitimate partner of the woman who had experienced a loss, delayed their own grieving in order to support their partners, and felt that healthcare providers were isolating. All of these sentiments and situations point to the gravidity that a pregnancy and subsequent loss has on the male partner in terms of his role as a husband, father, and a masculine figure (McCreight, 2004).

Gold et al. (2010) found a correlation between couples that experience pregnancy loss and shorter relationship survival rates. As partners are a main source of support for the woman in terms of her coping mechanisms, distress for either partner can lead to lower survival rates of relationships (Conway and Russell, 2000). This was true in Malissa's case, as she attributed her losses as a factor in her decision to no longer stay with her partner after her losses.

Conway and Russell (2000) also found that although both women and their partners experience distress immediately afterwards, the partners report feelings of sadness for longer periods of time. While there is some implementation of support for the women, there is no significant structure in place to help the partner with their own grief. This opposite to Susan's partner's experience when, "*he had to support me*". Unlike the study where the men had a delayed reaction, it was Susan who took a few weeks to really feel affected and her partner who was initially upset.

No matter how the stories of the women I talked to match up with specific study findings, it is evident how significantly relationships are altered by pregnancy loss. In "*Miscarriage Effects on Couples Interpersonal and Sexual Relationships During the First Year After Loss: Women's Perceptions*", Swanson et al. (2003) used qualitative perceptions of women who experienced miscarriages to analyze the influence of pregnancy loss on the relationship between partners. The study gave evidence that pregnancy loss changes the level of closeness in the relationship up to a year after loss, creates possible conflict in the between a woman and her partner, and exposes and magnifies difficulties that that may have existed prior to the pregnancy loss.

In addition to partners, research has also identified the more extended impact of pregnancy loss on overall social groups. Abboud et al. (2005) identified conflict with the types of coping strategies for the women, utilizing the partner as a main coping tool, the influence of gender roles in mourning, the role of family and friends, reactions from the community, the level of privacy around pregnancy loss, satisfaction with healthcare and providers, and the level of information made available. Rowsell et al. (2001) identified problems that arise when women with recurrent miscarriages utilize services for someone who has only had a single pregnancy loss because of the significantly different distress that this population experiences.

DeMontigny et al. (1999) used a qualitative study to further understand how a perinatal death affects the family and its relationship to its social network and overall support structure. In addition to results showing unsupportive, uneasy, and rushed reactions from healthcare providers, the researchers found that perinatal death profoundly affects a family's relationship and its support structures, possibly to the point of permanent change. There were several recurrent themes that matched up with the experiences of the women I talked to. For example, findings of unease with extended family members, and cultural perceptions that the pregnancy loss was not valid definitely occurred between Shannon and her in-laws. She felt that:

I am on good terms with my family but it's very stressful for me to be around my husband's family. I feel like they are very insensitive to the point of being cruel... After my first loss I felt like my husband and his family were very unsympathetic to my feelings. **Shannon**

Conflicts arise not only within the woman's own relationships to herself and her partner, but with her family, extended social networks, societal norms, healthcare structures, and provider sensitivity. The ramifications of involuntary pregnancy loss extend out to a large part of the community, magnify previous conflicts, leave the woman with a complex set of emotions, and expose the differences within communities.

The club no one wants to join

As I have come to find, with pregnancy loss you are either in or out. Women are talking about their experiences, but only within the pregnancy loss community. The women I talked to met me under the context of miscarriage. They set up a time with me and talked about their involuntary pregnancy loss. Then, twenty to forty-five minutes later, I disappeared and did not interfere with the other parts of their life. The only knowledge gained about me connected to what they personally experienced. Within this context, I was the perfect person to talk to:

> *Yeah I did that website...I used that a lot...I think those support groups that are on there were very helpful in healing because it's nice to have someone outside the family to talk to that...and they don't have any kind of judging; they don't know you, they don't know.* **Jenn**

That being said, you don't know until you know. It has been difficult approaching the inside world of involuntary pregnancy loss from the perspective of the outside. As Lisa explains:

> *I don't feel that someone who...I don't really feel like people who haven't experienced it can understand...you had kind of talked about 'can you speak to other people about it' and whatnot. But I really believe inside that it's the club no one wants to join. And you really...I don't really feel like I can have those conversations...those deep conversations about it with anybody else other than someone who has had the loss.* **Lisa**

Taking both of these ideas into account, my project is most useful when it is constructed as a link between the outside world and the

100

club no one wants to join. One has to recognize that you can listen, and you can support, but you can never really know. When you try to you run the risk of making the situation much worse:

People just don't understand so…that's very very difficult. And…people are just really really insensitive. They do not understand how to approach and what to say to a woman who has had a pregnancy loss, and just the things that come out of people's mouths! In fact, on my blog I even have a link to some like 'here's the stupid things people say'. Somewhere I include…all those things like 'you can have another' or 'well now that that's over' or you know? Just stupid things. **Lisa**

Jenni's experience casts light on what changes when you do join this community. I asked her how her feelings towards her sister, who had experienced an involuntary pregnancy loss before her, shifted once she herself had experienced one. She responded:

One of the things that I've experienced …is [that] you think of other people you know who had a pregnancy loss and you think 'oh my God was I there for that person, did I say anything dumb, did I take good care of them?' Because you don't really know fully what that pain is like or anything…like, 'was I just bitchy to my friend when she had a miscarriage'? **Jenni**

The Woodwork

What about interactions with other women who have experienced a miscarriage or a stillbirth? I was interested to find out how open the pregnancy loss community was once you have joined it. Several women answered this question with the same phrase:

No, but after people came out of the woodwork to tell me of their experiences or to mention someone they knew who had a miscarriage. **Shannon**

And I really…once you tell people that you have had a miscarriage, then people really come out of the woodwork. It just…it is so common. So there were a lot of people sharing their experiences with me. **Amy**

I didn't have any experience with pregnancy loss. But once I had a pregnancy loss women that I knew who had had losses told me that [about] losses that they hadn't told me [about] before. So there were several people that I knew that came out and told me that they had pregnancy losses. **Lisa**

Pregnancy loss is not so much a silent grief as it is a separate community. Most of the articles I read about silence and isolation during pregnancy loss portrayed a barren landscape where the only dialogue took place in the medical office. (Brier, 1999; Cote Arsenault et al., 2004) In reality, once you have found a vein, you are in the bloodline.

I am starting to understand the sentiment that generally one assumes they do not know women who have had pregnancy losses until they themselves experience it. This is evident in the narratives that Michael Berman (2001) presents in Parenthood Lost. Quite often women vocalized, " I used to think that pregnancy loss was something that happened to other people, not to me" (Berman, 2001:64-65). Then, suddenly, it seemed as if every woman in their life that they talk to had gone through it.

These experiences are ones that are burning to be told. What the medical and professional support community must realize is that trying to get women to open up about their experiences will not erode the silence around pregnancy loss. Connecting these women to each other and to an outlet where the memory can be shared will. After all, "only by listening to the full spectrum of stories that women confess to one another, including stories that they intuit they must not speak out loud in our culture, can the taboo against voicing our fears and bowdlerizing our experiences be broken" (Wolf, 2001:10).

If women who had experienced pregnancy loss felt comfortable talking to those who had not, perhaps the shift would not seem so drastic, and the community would not seem so invisible. But what would it take to change the tradition of only sharing your story with those who already know? What would it mean to open up to a community that not only has no idea what it feels like to have had a pregnancy loss but to be pregnant in the first place? How would people react to such a departure from a cultural norm?

Some of the answers to these questions lie in my own experience of entering a culture that I do not have a pass to. As well as enthusiasm, my interest in the topic of pregnancy loss and the telling of women's stories to alleviate silence has been met with surprise. During my research, I traveled to Virginia to attend the 2010 International Conference on Perinatal Loss and Infant death. The participants consisted of social workers, providers, nurses, and women who had themselves experienced a loss. Perhaps it was the difference of youth by a good ten years, or simply the fact that I definitely did not fit into any of these categories. Whatever it was, I caused a look of utter bewilderment on faces when I walked into presentations.

Another peculiar event has given me clues to these answers. Since starting the project on pregnancy loss, friends and family have tried to figure out the reason for my interest in the topic. Several people have asked me about my project, only to suddenly change the subject. Perhaps they all want to know if I am trying to end the silence on an experience I might have actually had. These interactions have made me realize several things. There may be no valid explanation for interest in such a topic if it does not directly apply to one's self. There also seems to be a significant level of withdrawal that occurs when such a taboo topic is thrown out onto the table. Finally, those who have had a pregnancy loss may ask the question as a preface to sharing a possible link. If a woman has not experienced a miscarriage, the significance of telling your own story would theoretically falter because you recognize your isolation in a shared experience and do not feel like you have a right to speak.

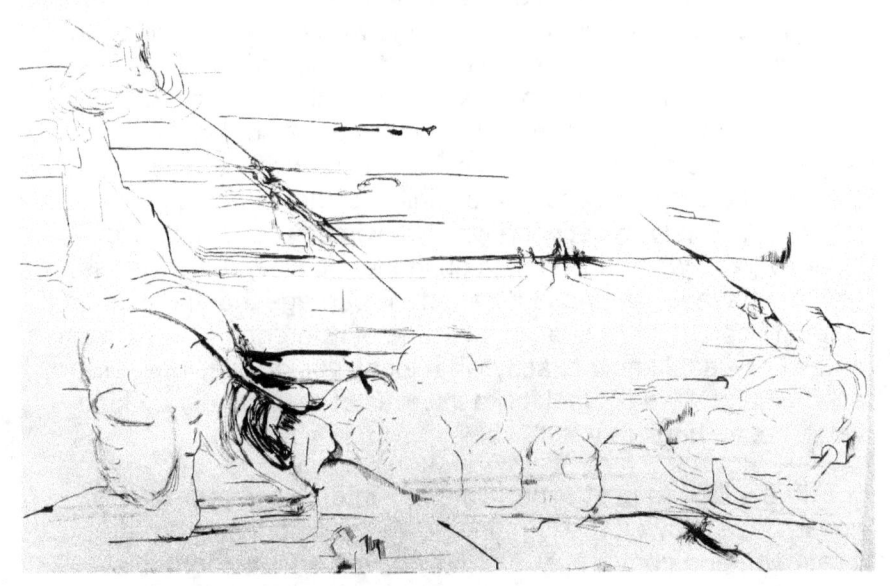

Part 3

Putting It Together

My position in the pregnancy loss community is unique in many ways. At first glance, it would appear that I possess all of the characteristics of an outsider. After all, I have to be aware that I am approaching this project as a young nulliparous college student who has no intention of getting pregnant or having children anytime soon. However, unlike many with that profile, I possess several unique viewpoints. Being the child of one who has lost a pregnancy, I am able to take the stance of a family member who lived through a miscarriage experience. Being the one who has seen some form of loss, my eyes have seen an expanded version of the darkness possible in life. I have not had personal bodily experience with pregnancy loss, but I have had the privilege of seeing the experience from the provider's point of view without having to assume the authority and responsibility of that role. I know what happens in the time between when a woman counts backwards from 100 and when she wakes up in the recovery room. In this sense, I have experienced a part of miscarriage that the women I talked to can't. There is a visual frame of reference when a woman dates her loss. I know exactly what eight weeks, twelve weeks, or even nineteen weeks looks like in terms of development. I know what those numbers entail. I also can't talk about it.

In addition to past experience, my interests in reproductive health have allowed me to gain knowledge about miscarriage, treatment, and community. Not only have I encountered the experiences of women who told me their stories, I have also sat down with providers, social workers, and researchers of miscarriage. Even having all of these perspectives is not adequate enough for me to understand or experience what the women I talked to went through. But they also prevent me from talking about or approaching the topic as a complete outsider. Instead, my combination of experience and non-experience puts me in a position to be able to bear witness to the stories and the experience of miscarriage rather than just listen.

It is important to note that all of the women in this study experienced losses of intended pregnancies. This factor may have significantly affected the ranges of experiences. For example, in a study by Beutel et al. (1995) women who had experienced wanted pregnancies reported significantly increased grief reactions. Although not all of the women who wanted their pregnancies experienced significant levels of grief, "the patients who had no measurable reaction to their miscarriage had never developed a strong attachment to their unborn child" (Beutel et al., 1995:525). This result is important. At the same time, it is also important to remember that each experience is individualized by its context. As Parsons (2010) describes it, "Women who miscarry have widely different responses to the experience: some find it life changing and mourn for years; others experience it as a momentary setback in their plans, or even as a relief" (6).

From what I could gather from the miscarriage literature, most involuntary losses are assumed to be wanted pregnancies. However, this idea is not a fact so much as a historical remnant. In her analysis of how miscarriage was publicly represented in the 20th century, Reagan (2003) found that "...when articles about miscarriage first appeared in popular women's magazines during the 1940's, they all assumed that miscarriage represented the loss of wanted children to married couples" (361). This evidence implies that the reasons behind these assumptions in the present day are simply cultural norms that were put in place in the 1940's. As there has been no cultural or political impetus to change this type of thinking, the assumption stayed. And the longer it did, the more it appeared to be a fact rather than a culturally produced theory.

If all losses are assumed to be intended pregnancies, it makes sense that the literature also assumes significant sadness. Currently, "...in the United States, women are expected to grieve their miscarriages" (Reagan, 2003:359). However, In contrast to assumptions about intended pregnancies, grief was not always an expectation. Historically, "although midcentury political writers recognized the unhappiness ...following miscarriage...they did not emphasize grief" (Reagan, 2003:361). The pro family culture of the 1940's and 50's focused mainly on trying again for more children and was the most likely reason that grief was not publicized.

At what point did the public expectation about the miscarriage experience shift? Starting in the 1970's, the pregnancy loss movement was taken up by mainly middle class white women. According to Reagan (2003), this resulted in the expectation "...to grieve-in a ritualized and public format..." (366). Although each woman I talked to had individual reasons for the outcome of her experience, it is safe to say that public expectations of sadness might have played a role in how they vocalized these sentiments to me.

Even if one is taking an objective stance towards cultural norms, one must be careful not to forget that such a project will inevitably face these constraints. There is no other legitimate frame of reference. In her anthropological critique of fetal rationality in feminist philosophy, Morgan (1996) found that "we have a responsibility to formulate responses with a heightened awareness to the historical and cultural idiosyncrasies of those traditions, and to make our reflexivity explicit" (62). To approach a project with the assumption that it is not interconnected with social and historical aspects is to be irresponsible.

In spite of my attempts at reflexive awareness, I came into my thesis with quite a few assumptions. I was sure that miscarriage was never discussed. On the other hand, I was positive the event significantly impacted the life of any woman it touched in the same way. I expected that the scientific literature completely and comprehensively analyzed and understood the experience. And I was sure that reading enough about it would completely prepare me for what I would hear. Rather than new knowledge, the stories I found would only serve as detail and evidence.

That was wrong. By the middle of my project, I had started to accept that any assumption I ever made would be contradicted. Keeping this context in mind, I came out of my interviews and analysis with several questions, challenges to established wisdom, and new thoughts: that science's subjectivity in assuming objectivity limits its abilities; that other children make a significant impact on the overall experience; that the miscarriage experience is not silenced so much as segregated; and that it all comes down to perceptions of control.

Approaching a culture of no culture

The problem with science is its propensity to deny its own imperfections. Such a perceived objectivity and lack of opinion is in and of itself a culture of no culture. In her essay on the topic, Janelle Taylor (2003) defines this paradox as "a community defined by the shared cultural conviction that its shared convictions were not in the least cultural, but, rather, timeless truths" (556). To assume a lack of cultural norms in scientific literature is in itself a cultural norm. The studies I read on miscarriage took a very objective stance towards the women's emotions and reactions. However, being objective is a cultural aspect of research, therefore it can be considered biased. Taking this into account, perhaps my assumptions about the perfection of evidence based research were not a result of my forgetfulness so much as an understanding based within the context of my culture.

The culture of no culture may mean that some inaccuracies stem from a lack of categorization. When it comes to miscarriage, nothing can be done to reverse the process and there is no definite category in which to place the experience. They "...are seen as neither illness nor injury, neither a life to be saved nor a death to be mourned" (Reinharz, 1988:88). If the goal of modern medicine is to fix what is broken, putting time and energy into something that is neither fixable nor definite is seen as a waste of resources. This idea is additionally reflected in the shift involved in viewing miscarriage as a possible and common outcome of pregnancy to that of an unexplained anomaly.

Other children

Another important aspect of the miscarriage experience is that it occurs in a spectrum of reproductive occurrences rather than simply by itself. Other life factors must therefore be taken into account. One of the most significant realizations I had over the course of my interviews involved the importance of children. In doing my preliminary research for this project, I had seen information on the topic, but did not give it much thought. My focus had been on the pregnancy losses at hand, not the successful reproductive occurrences that preceded or followed it. After concluding my interviews and really taking a moment to look at what the women had collectively shown me, I went back and refocused on what had seemed so trivial. What I found the second time around is a good indicator of how easy it is to selectively choose what we take away from data in research.

Although there have been some varying results, for the most part, the literature leaned towards the theory that other children make all the difference in the level of emotional distress the women experience after an involuntary pregnancy loss (Brier, 2008; Cote-Arsenault and Mahlangu, 1998; Fertl et al., 2009; Neugebaur et al.,

1992; Swanson et al., 2007). Some of this research focused on the positive effects that the presence of children had. Neugebauer et al. (1992) found no significant increase in the symptoms of distress for women with children who had recently experienced a miscarriage and the control group (women who had not been pregnant in the past year, though some had experienced reproductive losses and half had living biological children). Other research focused on the negative effects that childlessness had on the miscarriage experience. In their review of this literature, Brier (2008) found that "Studies related to the absence of living children at the time of miscarriage seem consistent in indicating relatively higher levels of grief in women who do not have living children" (460). In their review of two studies that looked at the effect of childlessness on the experience of miscarriage, Klier et al. (2002) found that "...the overall effect of miscarriage was substantially worse among childless women...for major depressive disorder in particular, the relative risk was substantially higher for childless women..." (137).

It is obvious from my interview results and my double reading of the scientific literature that living children serve as a buffer to negative aspects of the miscarriage experience. The question is why this has such a significant effect. Some of the researchers gave short explanations for their results. For women who had positive correlations, Neugebauer et al. (1992) concluded that children were effective in reducing symptoms because they represented "...evidence of reproductive success in the past" (1338). For women who did not have children, Fertl et al. (2009) proposed that increased grief stems from "A more intense fear of never having children or more children..." (26).

In addition to living children, researchers also applied these cultural theories to explain a childless woman's anxiety to become pregnant again. For example, Swanson et al. (2007) theorized "For some childless women, a miscarriage...might leave childless women anxious about their ability to ever bear children" (14). The experience for women who do not yet have children carries very different connotations than for those who do. Nagel (2004) found that "if the fetus dies, her [the woman's] status as a mother is...challenged" (233). If there is no living evidence to prove a woman's reproductive success, she does not possess the ability to claim motherhood. Although having a subsequent successful pregnancy and child would not fill the loss, it would allow her to officially and publicly call herself   a mother.

There is a universal expectation to redeem oneself after a miscarriage. For a childless woman, society views the loss as part of the path to parenthood rather than a separate event. Infertility as a whole is a culturally defined as a space between. "...It is a condition of not yet achieving or maintaining a viable pregnancy...thus infertility seems like a tentative condition until all one's options have run out" (Chase and Rogers, 2001:175). This adds to the expectation that the miscarriage will not be mourned or considered permanent. When a childless woman who has experienced a loss does not attempt a subsequent pregnancy, there are social consequences. Reinharz (1988) found that "as long as the potential to conceive remains, miscarriage is likely to be considered a small loss. Thus, if a woman defines her loss as real, large or permanent, she may be perceived as unreasonable" (89).

All of these results left me wondering where the cultural expectation to prove one's capability comes from. Whereas the studies I read focused on the effect of having children on depression, grief, and anxiety, I was interested in how this factor could possibly create feelings of guilt and failure. There is a connection between having children, needing to prove the ability to do so, and the guilt and blame that one commonly experiences if they can't. For example, Klier et al. (2002) conducted an extensive review of the literature and found that for women without children, miscarriage "...may produce doubts about procreative competence. As a consequence, miscarriage may increase women's risk for psychiatric symptoms and disorders" (129). The reasons may stem from the cultural and historical factors of what reproduction encompasses, how it influences, and whom it benefits. Women who experience a miscarriage may feel a sense of failure because the loss represents a flaw within them. The individual experience also reflects on the collective ability. For example, Diamond and Seidenberg (1995) found that "the notion that the health of individual bodies is related to the health of the social body..." (90). If an individual has a utilitarian responsibility to do what is best for the community and an individual's actions reflect the actions of the entire community, a miscarriage would mean that the individual failed the community as well as themselves.

Reproductive expectations also stem from cultural responsibility. One is expected to participate in society through the production of something beneficial. If Ginsberg and Rapp (1991) were correct that American culture views children as "flawless commodities", then the ability to produce such currency would be the perfect societal participation. Women who feel guilty because they are unable to create this commodity confuse responsibility with culpability (Hale, 2007). Whereas responsibility is defined as "fulfilling one's duty" culpability can be interpreted as "deserving blame" (Hale, 2007:25). In his explanation of the distinction between the two, Hale (2007) found that "When the chosen route...does not lead where we thought it would lead, it is easy to imagine that we have failed in our responsibility and that we are therefore culpable" (25).

A part of blame is the assumption that the person who has failed could have chosen a different outcome. For example, women may feel that their eating, sleeping, and exercise habits contributed to the loss of the pregnancy. Much emphasis is placed on women to have a healthy pregnancy and as a result a miscarriage may be seen as proof that they were not living in the right way. Parsons (2010) cites Layne's (2003) theory that:

> In the United States we tend to understand moral stature and worldly success to be the result of purposeful, individual effort, a reproductive 'failure' like pregnancy loss is often understood by women to be somehow their fault. Although physicians routinely reassure women post facto that there was nothing they could have done to cause their loss, this message contradicts all of the morally laden messages they have received throughout the pregnancy regarding their personal responsibility for the well being of their child (Parsons, 2010:20).

Blaming the woman's miscarriage on her habits and behaviors may create a need to "redeem" ones self after the experience. A subsequent successful pregnancy enables the woman to prove that she has now made the correct choices in terms of her behavior.

Klier et al. (2002) found that that if a subsequent pregnancy also ends in a loss, grief reactions are significantly increased. However, Malpas and Solomon (1998) theorized that people would often risk the experience of pain in order to gain control of the situation. (26) Basic motivation to redeem oneself therefore outweighs the risk of further loss and sadness. This would explain the high rate of pregnancies after an initial loss. Klier et al. (2002) also cites a sample group in which "over 86 percent of 221 women who lost a child by miscarriage (approximately 85 percent) or perinatal death (approximately 15 percent) conceived again within a year and a half following loss…the majority of women (63 percent) were pregnant again at six months following loss" (140). Control may even be part of the reason for increased grief. As Parsons (2010) found, "Sometimes crying, sadness, and depression after a miscarriage might be attributable more to the loss of control a woman feels over her body or over her plans for the future, than grief over the death of the embryo/fetus itself" (15).

Miscarriage as a segregated experience

It is very easy to proclaim the need for open dialogue about miscarriage and involuntary pregnancy loss. Sitting down with women and asking them to tell you their story seems very simple, as does the project of finding concrete, universal themes that all women who go through a miscarriage experience. Such a project, however, would get no one anywhere fast.

From what I could tell, research theories about pregnancy loss assume that if women open up about their experience, all cultural stigmas around it will cease. I think it would probably help. However, I also think that if simply breaking the silence could solve the entire problem, most conflicts around miscarriage and involuntary pregnancy loss would have been fixed a long time ago. What we need to acknowledge is that it *is* being talked about. There is a community- in support groups, on online message boards, and at kitchen tables. Women are talking. The problem is, very few of their family members, friends, and communities are listening.

It is easy to say that I was welcomed into the community. I was. I sat through the lectures, met with the leaders of loss groups, and listened to women tell me their stories. However, at no point was I a member. Rather, I filled the role of the outsider who wanted to bear witness. And that's exactly where I wanted to be. I would suggest that the silence of the miscarriage experience can only be broken if we also disrupt the barrier between the involuntary pregnancy loss community and everyone else.

Dialogue and information within the miscarriage community needs to be introduced into the public eye. However, I have concerns about the effect that mainstreaming the pregnancy loss community would have on its support structure and abilities. If Lisa is correct that you can never fully understand unless you have experienced it, then opening up the community to everyone would erode the kind of "I've been there" honesty and possibly the only support that some women have.

"Breaking the silence" has been attempted without the context of an acknowledged lack of awareness. And it usually goes horribly wrong. For example, one only has to look on the pregnancy loss blogs (such as Lisa's) for "Stupid Things People Say." To be useful and supportive, breaking the silence has to be much more specific. What needs to be broken is the silence of information. This also is easier said than done. As Lexi said, "*Who is going to sponsor the website about dead babies? Not the formula companies.*" For silence to be broken, cultural norms need to shift. And for norms to shift, there needs to be either a major cultural disruption or an incentive.

At first glance, "breaking the silence" appears to be a valid solution. However, it can only be effective if the change it creates includes a dialogue between the involuntary pregnancy loss community and everyone else. However, opening up this dialogue can only be successful under a few conditions: those of us trying to understand the experience through an objective and empathetic point of view must listen to these stories with the understanding that knowing does not mean experiencing; it means bearing witness. We may not be part of the pregnancy loss community, but chances are someone who is very important in our life is. A lot of these women are mothers, sisters, and aunts. They are definitely daughters. Approaching miscarriage through the connections that we have with those who have experienced it allows us to create a strong support network for these individuals.

If one attempts to bear witness only through listening, the burden of being educated about involuntary pregnancy loss falls back on to that community. In order to bear witness actively, we must also educate ourselves about the topic. And as a daughter of one who has lost several pregnancies, I can tell you this: what holds us back from discussing and learning about involuntary pregnancy loss also holds us back from everything else. Once the intimate barrier of letting someone in on your own personal thoughts is broken, the relationship as a whole shifts.

Life, death, and politics

For women, physicians, activists, and the general public, miscarriage represents an uncomfortable proximity to the apex between life and death. There are two cultural ways to approach these states. They can be seen as either opposite ends of the spectrum or as connecting points in a cycle (Malpas and Solomon, 1998). Western culture generally defines birth and pregnancy as the opposite of dying and death. However, I agree with the opinion that defining "…birth without acknowledging the familiar presence of death as attendant seems like those contemporary half experiences: safer, cleaner, wholly more desirable, yet somehow not quite real" (Wolf, 2001:80). Miscarriage negates the security of birth being "safer" and "cleaner" because it is a state of transition. It has the capability to remind us that pregnancy is a possible path to death or life, rather than a definite means to the latter.

It is also this association that pulls miscarriage into the political arena of abortion. Many would argue that acknowledging miscarriage as a death implies the acknowledgement of pregnancy as a life, which would define the loss as the deprivation of life. But if life is contingent upon the act of possessing self-identity and awareness (Malpas and Solomon, 1998) then something that is not autonomous cannot lose its sense of self. Miscarriage is not the death of something that was once alive; rather it is the death of a possibility. To some women, they are losing a baby, but to many others they are losing the chance for a baby.

Many of the feminist texts on pregnancy loss that I have come across criticize the reproductive rights movement for staying away from pregnancy loss support because of these possible connections to the pro-life movement (Layne, 2003). However, this may be the reason that involuntary pregnancy loss support sometimes falls into the pro-life lane. One of the reasons that the involuntary pregnancy loss support movement only " draws on the anti-abortion movement and feminism to comprehend and define miscarriage…" (Reagan, 2003:359) is because there is no other movement to draw on. If the reproductive rights and abortion rights movements do not acknowledge involuntary pregnancy loss as a significant event, they cannot influence its support structures.

Other reasons for pro-life sentiments may lie in the limited language available to describe the experience. As Reagan (2003) reminds readers, "the terms *baby* and *abortion* are value-laden and highly contested" (358). Both Layne (2001) and Reagan (2003) also found "use of the anti-abortion movement's language in *official* hospital materials" (Reagan, 2003:367). Use of words such as "baby", and imagery such as footprints may be important to some women. To others, however, it places their loss in the context of a movement that they are against. As an abortion rights advocate, it was difficult at times for me to navigate my own narrative in ways that did not use pro-life language. However, there was no other language available to use.   Additionally, some of the women I talked to did consider their miscarriages to be a loss not only of a baby, but their baby. Had I not decided write about their experiences in the language that they themselves specifically utilized, my disrespect and bias would had taken precedent over their experience. I am simultaneously an abortion activist and the daughter of a woman with very pro-life beliefs. Although I am definite about what side of the spectrum I am on, I am also aware that my actions would be identical to someone who was pro-life if I perceived pregnancy and birth as they did. This allows me to approach the topic with the understanding that many others do not hold my views.

This situation left me in conflict. How would I create a narrative that respected the words and beliefs of others without accidentally using a framework I fundamentally disagreed with? For me, the best way to differentiate between abortion and miscarriage was to define the former as a choice to not self-identify and the latter as the loss of chosen self-identification. It is up to the woman to decide whether or not to consider her pregnancy part of herself. In cases of abortion where the pregnancy is not wanted, there is often no self-identification. Rather, the pregnancy is seen as an event that is separate both from the woman and the possibility of a baby. In the cases of miscarriage where the woman's pregnancy has taken on these characteristics, there is much more to lose in terms of possibility.

Another major difference between the two events casts light on a realization I had after my interviews. When it comes down to it, how a woman experiences her miscarriage is a matter of perceived control. Swanson et al.'s (2007) review of the current literature on women's responses to miscarriage found that women report among other symptoms, a "lack of control" (4). Callander et al. (2007) also cites a study finding that women may feel a need to regain control during the miscarriage experience and that this need may cause behavioral changes after the miscarriage. Control would explain the significant effect of other children on the experience, as success is an indicator of autonomy. Additionally, control would explain the issues around the use of the word 'miscarriage', as the word defines the loss as a result of helplessness. Finally, it would explain why the miscarriage community is so hidden. In separating itself from the mainstream, the women in the miscarriage community can maintain a sense of control over support and information about the experience even if it cannot control the event itself.

Reflections

This project has been one of the most challenging experiences I have ever willingly put myself through. Miscarriage, loss, and grief were the only things I seemingly thought about, talked about, and read about for months. My biggest question through all of it was "why am I doing this to myself?" Why not choose to focus my attention, energy, and culmination of all of my work on something happy? Why bring sadness into my every day life voluntarily?

My work did seriously affect me, and not necessarily in a completely positive way. I am proud to look back and see that I taught myself about a life experience I previously wasn't aware existed, and I went into the community to see for myself. I am not so proud that I let this attempt almost completely consume me. It is a very difficult thing to spend your days in the grief of others without bringing those stories home with you. It is even harder to not let those stories replace your own. My biggest struggle throughout my work was how to place the information I had in the context of my own life rather than letting it control my entire life's context. Making room in my head for the experiences of twelve women caused me, in some ways, to lose my own.

Or even more than a little bit. As I got deeper and deeper into my work, I started to notice how my knowledge was fine-tuning the factors in the rest of my life. Every action and event I encountered became situated on a scale I had created to judge how much control was at stake and who had it. When I encountered moments of

116

sadness or misfortune for others, it was almost as if I had reached my empathy saturation point. I didn't want to hear about it, I had listened enough.

An experience towards the end of my rough draft woke me up to the fact that in listening to others I had stopped listening to myself. It also highlighted the importance of a support system that relies on shared experience. I had been convinced to go to a group on bereavement that someone at my college had started even though it was not the first meeting. I finally decided to go in an effort to seek sense of shared experience. A friend mentioned that everyone who had come to the group had done so as a result of losing a father. I told her I would check it out, and spent the rest of the day deciding if I needed to. After all, my father had passed away two years ago; bereaved was no longer a synonym for me. In my mind, I had mourned, gotten on with life, and had moved on. I didn't think such a place would do me any good.

When I got to the room, I was fine. I sat down, the door was closed, and everyone started to go around with introductions. I was the last one to speak, and was completely fine for the words "My name is". Then I paused and realized that this moment was the first time I had ever been in a room where the only shared experience was the one that I had never been able to share. Perhaps it was a result of hearing it over and over again from so many texts and women. Perhaps it was the ability to let my guard down. Perhaps it was nothing but what it was. Regardless, the floodgates opened. I am eternally grateful to the women who contacted me, met with me, picked up the phone, and talked. Until that moment in that room, I had been grateful that they were willing to share their story. Now I am grateful that they had shared their stories in spite of how easy it is not to. It seemingly takes no effort in this world to not speak up. If you have experienced the feeling of falling, there is a natural hesitation to risk losing control another time. I want to thank these women regardless of whether their experience is one that they would categorize as sad or significant. I also want to acknowledge my respect for these women who opened up to me even though I did not share a common experience. To tell of loss without the assurance that those listening have also felt grief is hard. But Lisa, Jennifer, Cindy, Jenn, Susan, Jenni, Amy, Lexi, Malissa, Amber, Shannon and Kirsten did it anyway.

Part 1: Works Cited

Abboud, L., and Liamputtong, P. "When pregnancy fails: coping strategies, support networks and experiences with health care of ethnic women and their partners." *Journal of Reproductive & Infant Psychology* 23.1 (2005): 3-18.

Alizade, A. (Ed.). *Motherhood in the Twenty-first Century*. London: Karnac, 2006. Print.

Bowles, S., et al. "Acute and post-traumatic stress disorder after spontaneous abortion." *American Family Physician*, (2000): 1-9.

Chase, S., and Rogers, M. *Mothers and Children: Feminist Analysis and Personal Narratives*. London: Rutgers University Press, 2001. Print.

Collins, J., and David, R."Birth weight among infants of U.S.-born blacks, African-born blacks, and U.S.-born whites." *New Engl J Med* 337 (1997): 1209-1214.

Côte-Arsenault, D., et al. "Support groups helping women through pregnancies after loss." *West J Nurs Res* 26.6 (2004): 650-670.

De Montigny, F., Beaudet, L., and Dumas, L. "A baby has died: the impact of perinatal loss on family social networks." *Journal of Obstetrics, Gynecologic, and Neonatal Nursing* 28.2 (1999):151-56.

Farquharson, R., Jauniaux, E., and Exalto, N., "Updated and revised nomenclature for description of early pregnancy events." *Human Reproduction* 20 (2005): 3008-3011.

Freudenberg N., and Ruglis, J., "Reframing school dropout as a public health issue." *Prev Chronic Dis* 4.4 (2007): 1-11.

Getz, D. "Men's and Women's Earnings for States and Metropolitan Statistical Areas: 2009." Issue brief no. 09/3. *American Community Survey*. Print.

Kirsch, I, et al. "Adult Literacy in America: A First Look at the Findings of the National Adult Literacy Survey". Rep. no.

1993-275. 3rd ed. National Center for Education Statistics, (2002) Print.

La Rochebrochard, E., and Thonneau, P. "Paternal age and maternal age are risk factors for miscarriage: results of a multicenter European study." *Human Reproduction*. 17.6 (2002): 1649-1656.

Lanthrop, M. "Affirming Motherhood: Lessons from Mothers' Narratives of Perinatal   Hospice." Diss. Marquette University, 2009. Print. Presented at the 2010 International Conference on Perinatal and Infant Death in Alexandria, Virginia.

Layne, L. Motherhood Lost: a Feminist Account of Pregnancy Loss in America. New York: Routledge, 2003. Print.

Neugebauer, R., et al. "Association of stressful life events with chromosomally normal spontaneous abortion." *American Journal of Epidemiology* 143.6 (1996): 588-596.

Nielsen, S., et al. "Bereavement, grieving, and psychological morbidity after first trimester spontaneous abortion: comparing expectant management with surgical evaluation." *Human Reproduction,* 11.8 (1996): 1767-1770.

Nikčević, A.V. "Development and evaluation of a miscarriage follow-up clinic." *Journal of Reproductive & Infant Psychology* 21.3 (2003): 207-217.

Parazzini, F., et al. "Determinants of risk of spontaneous abortions in the first trimester of pregnancy." *Epidemiology* 8.6 (1997): 681-683.

Price, S. "Prevalence and Correlation of Pregnancy Loss History in a National Sample of Children and Families." *Maternal and Child Health Journal* 10 (2006): 489-500.

Reagan, L. "From hazard to blessing to tragedy: representations of miscarriage in twentieth century America." *Feminist Studies* 29.2 (2003):356-378.

Reinharz, S. "What's missing in miscarriage?" *Journal of Community Psychology*. 16.1 (1988): 84-103.

Rich, A. *Of Woman Born: Motherhood as Experience and Institution*. New York: Norton, 1976. Print.

Swanson, K., et al. "Contexts and evolution of women's responses to miscarriage during the first year after loss." *Research in Nursing and Health* 30 (2007): 2-16.

Sumrall, A., and Vecchione, P. *Catholic Girls*. New York, NY: Penguin, 1992. Print.

U.S Census Bureau. *Population Distribution and Change: 2000 to 2010*. Issue brief. Print. 2010 Census Briefs.

Van, P. "Breaking the silence of African American women: healing after pregnancy loss." *Health Care for Women International* 22.3 (2001): 229-243.

Ventura, S., et al. *Estimated Pregnancy Rates by Outcome for the United States, 1990–2004*. Center for Disease Control, 56.12 (2008)

Weck, R., et al. "Impact on environmental factors and poverty on pregnancy outcomes." *Clinical Obstetrics and Gynecology* 51.2 (2008): 349-359.

Weitz, R. *The Politics of Women's Bodies: Sexuality, Appearance, and Behavior*. New York: Oxford UP, 2003. Print.

Milestones: Works Cited

Abboud, L., and Liamputtong, P. "When pregnancy fails: coping strategies, support networks and experiences with health care of ethnic women and their partners." *Journal of Reproductive & Infant Psychology* 23.1 (2005): 3-18.

Adolfsson, A., et al. "Guilt and emptiness: women's experiences with miscarriage." *Health Care for Women International* 25.6 (2004): 542-560.

Klier, C. et al. "Affective disorders in the aftermath of miscarriage: A comprehensive review." *Archives of Women's Mental Health*, 5 (2002): 129-149.

Kowaleski J. *State definitions and reporting requirements for live births, fetal deaths, and induced terminations of pregnancy (1997 revision).* Hyattsville, Maryland: National Center for Health Statistics. 1997.

Michels, T., and Tiu, A. "Second Trimester Pregnancy Loss." *American Family Physician* 76.9 (2007): 1341-346.

"Miscarry - Definition and More from the Free Merriam-Webster Dictionary." *Merriam-Webster Online*. Web. 16 Nov. 2010.

Neugebauer, R., et al. "Association of stressful life events with chromosomally normal spontaneous abortion." *American Journal of Epidemiology* 143.6 (1996): 588-596.

Rai, R., and Regan, L., "Recurrent miscarriage." *The Lancet* 368.9535 (2006): 601-611.

Scott, J. (ed.) *Danforth's Obstetrics and Gynecology* 8th ed. Philadelphia: Lippincott, Williams & Wilkins, 1999.

Seri, I., and Evans, J. "Limits of viability: definition of the gray zone." *Journal of Perinatology* 28 (2008): S4-8.

Sonstegard, Lois J., Karren Mundell. Kowalski, and Betty Jennings. *Women's Health*. New York: Grune & Stratton, 1983. Print.

"Spontaneous Abortion." Word Net. Miriam Webster. Web. 21 Nov. 2010.

Swanson, K., Connor, S., Jolley, S., et al. "Contexts and evolution of women's responses to miscarriage during the first year after loss." *Research in Nursing and Health* 30 (2007): 2-16.

Wright, P. "Pushing On: A Grounded Theory Study of Maternal Perinatal Bereavement." Diss. Scranton University, 2010. Print. Presented at the 2010 International Conference on Perinatal and Infant Death in Alexandria, Virginia.

Power: Works Cited

Chambers, G, and Sullivan, E. "The Economic Impact of Assisted Reproductive Technology: A Review of Selected Developed Countries." *Fertility and Sterility* 91.6 (2009): 2281-2294.

Cottingham, J. *A Descartes Dictionary*. Oxford, OX, UK: Blackwell Reference, 1993. Print.

Joraleman, Donald. "The Healer's Role." ANT-248 Medical Anthropology Class. Smith College, Northampton. 2 Mar. 2010. Lecture. Notes from lecture are cited.

Layne, Linda L. Motherhood Lost: a Feminist Account of Pregnancy Loss in America. New York: Routledge, 2003. Print.

Levy, A., and Widra., E. "Basic Infertility: Etiology and Therapy." *The Physiologic Basis of Gynecology and Obstetrics,* 2001. Print.

McCracken, Elizabeth. *An Exact Replica of a Figment of My Imagination: a Memoir*. New York: Little, Brown and, 2008. Print.
Reagan, L. "From Hazard to Blessing to Tragedy: Representations of Miscarriage in Twentieth-Century America." Feminist Studies 29.2 (2003):356-378.

Rich, Adrienne Cecile. *Of Woman Born: Motherhood as Experience and Institution*. New York: Norton, 1976. Print.

Schieve, L., et al. "Spontaneous Abortion Among Pregnancies Conceived Using Assisted Reproductive Technology in the United States." Obstetrics and Gynecology 101.5 (2003):959-967.

Scott, J. (ed.) *Danforth's Obstetrics and Gynecology* 8th ed. Philadelphia: Lippincott, Williams & Wilkins, 1999.

Pain: Works Cited

Abboud, L., and Liamputtong, P. "When pregnancy fails: coping strategies, support networks and experiences with health care of ethnic women and their partners." *Journal of*

Reproductive & Infant Psychology 23.1 (2005): 3-18.

Adolfsson, A., et al. ""Guilt and emptiness: women's experiences with miscarriage."" *Health Care for Women International* 25.6 (2004):542-560.

Bansen, S., and Stevens, H. "Women's experiences of miscarriage in early pregnancy." *Journal of Nurse-Midwifery* 37.2 (1992):84-90.

Berman, M. *Parenthood Lost: Healing the Pain after Miscarriage, Stillbirth, and Infant Death.* Westport, CT: Bergin & Garvey, 2001. Print.

Brier, N. "Clinical Commentary: Understanding and managing the emotional reactions to a miscarriage." *Obstetrics and Gynecology* 93.1 (1999): 151-155.

Martin, E. *The Woman in the Body: a Cultural Analysis of Reproduction.* Boston: Beacon, 2001. Print.

Reagan, L. "From Hazard to Blessing to Tragedy: Representations of Miscarriage in Twentieth-Century America." Feminist Studies 29.2 (2003):356-378.

Scott, J. (ed.) *Danforth's Obstetrics and Gynecology* 8th ed. Philadelphia: Lippincott, Williams & Wilkins, 1999.

Swanson, K., et al. "Contexts and Evolution of Women's Responses to Miscarriage During the First Year after Loss." Research in Nursing & Health 30 (2007): 2-16.

Wright, P. "Pushing On: A Grounded Theory Study of Maternal Perinatal Bereavement." Diss. Scranton University, 2010. Print. Presented at the 2010 International Conference on Perinatal and Infant Death in Alexandria, Virginia.

Stigma: Works Cited

Adolfsson, A., et al. ""Guilt and emptiness: women's experiences with miscarriage."" *Health Care for Women International* 25.6 (2004):542-560.

Berman, M. *Parenthood Lost: Healing the Pain after Miscarriage, Stillbirth, and Infant Death*. Westport, CT: Bergin & Garvey, 2001. Print.

Davis-Floyd, R. *Birth as an American Rite of Passage*. Berkeley: University of California, 2003. Print.

Layne, L. *Motherhood Lost: a Feminist Account of Pregnancy Loss in America*. New York: Routledge, 2003. Print.

Kluger-Bell, K. *Unspeakable Losses: Understanding the Experience of Pregnancy Loss, Miscarriage, and Abortion*. New York: W.W. Norton, 1998. Print.

McCracken, E. *An Exact Replica of a Figment of My Imagination: a Memoir*. New York: Little, Brown and, 2008. Print.

St. John, A.,et al. "Shrouds of silence: three women's stories of prenatal loss."*Australian Journal of Advanced Nursing,* 23.3 (2006): 8-12.

Weitz, Rose. *The Politics of Women's Bodies: Sexuality, Appearance, and Behavior*. New York: Oxford UP, 2003. Print.

Distance: Works Cited

Abboud, L., and Liamputtong, P. "When pregnancy fails: coping strategies, support networks and experiences with health care of ethnic women and their partners." Journal of Reproductive & Infant Psychology 23.1 (2005): 3-18.

Berman, M. *Parenthood Lost: Healing the Pain after Miscarriage, Stillbirth, and Infant Death*. Westport, CT: Bergin & Garvey, 2001. Print.

Brier, N. "Clinical Commentary: Understanding and managing the emotional reactions to a miscarriage." *Obstetrics and Gynecology* 93.1 (1999): 151-155.

Conway, K., and Russell, G. "Couples' grief and experience of support in the aftermath of miscarriage." British Journal of Medical Psychology 73.4 (2000): 531-545.

Côte-Arsenault, D., et al. "Support groups helping women through pregnancies after loss." West J Nurs Res 26.6 (2004): 650-670.

"De Montigny, F., Beaudet, L., and Dumas, L. ""A baby has died: the impact of perinatal loss on family social networks."" *Journal of Obstetrics, Gynecologic, and Neonatal Nursing,* 28.2 (1999): 151-56.

"Gold, K., et al. "Marriage and cohabitation outcomes after pregnancy loss." *Pediatrics,* 25.5 (2010): e1202-e1207.

Klier, C. et al. "Affective disorders in the aftermath of miscarriage: A comprehensive review." *Archives of Women's Mental Health,* 5 (2002): 129-149.

Mcreight, S. "A grief ignored: narratives of pregnancy loss from a male perspective." *Sociology of Health and Illness,* 26.3 (2004): 326-350.

Nikčević, A.V. "Development and evaluation of a miscarriage follow-up clinic." *Journal of Reproductive & Infant Psychology* 21.3 (2003): 207.

Rowsell, E., et al. "The psychological impact of recurrent miscarriage, and the role of counselling at a pre-pregnancy counseling clinic." *Journal of Reproductive & Infant Psychology* 19.1 (2001): 33-45.

Swanson, K., et al. "Miscarriage effects on couples' interpersonal and sexual relationships during the first year after loss: women's perceptions." *Psychosomatic Medicine,* 65 (2003): 902-910.

Wolf, N. *Misconceptions: Truth, Lies, and the Unexpected on the Journey to Motherhood.* New York: Doubleday, 2001. Print.

Part 3:Works Cited

Beutel, M., et al. "Grief and depression after miscarriage: their separation, antecedents, and course." *Psychosomatic Medicine,* 57 (1995): 517-526.

Brier, N. "Grief following miscarriage: a comprehensive review of the literature." *Journal of Women's Health,* 17.3 (2008): 451-464.

Callander, G., et al. "Counterfactual thinking and psychological distress following recurrent miscarriage." *Journal of Reproductive & Infant Psychology* 25.1 (2007): 51-65.

Chase, S., and Rogers, M. *Mothers and Children: Feminist Analysis and Personal Narratives.* London: Rutgers University Press, 2001. Print.

Cote-Arsenault, D., and Mahlangu, N. "Impact of perinatal loss on the subsequent pregnancy and self: women's experiences." *JOGNN,* 28.3 (1998): 274-282.

Diamond, I., and Seidenberg, D. "Review: Embracing mystery: Fertile Ground: Women, Earch, and the Limits of Control." *Bridges,* 5.2 (1995): 90-91.

Fertl, K., et al. "Levels and effects of different forms of anxiety during pregnancy after a prior miscarriage." *European Journal of Obstetrics and Gynecology and Reproductive Biology,* 142.1 (2009): 23-29.

Ginsberg, F., and Rapp, R. "The politics of reproduction." *Annual Review of Anthropology,* 20 (1991): 311-343.

Hale, B. "Culpability and blame after pregnancy loss." *Journal of Medical Ethics,* 33 (2007): 24-27.

Klier, C. et al. "Affective disorders in the aftermath of miscarriage: A comprehensive review." *Archives of Women's Mental Health,* 5 (2002): 129-149.

Layne, L. *Motherhood Lost: a Feminist Account of Pregnancy Loss in America.* New York: Routledge, 2003. Print.

Malpas, J., and Solomon, R. *Death and Philosophy.* London: Routledge, 1998. Print.

Morgan, L. "Fetal rationality in feminist philosophy: an anthropological critique." *Hypatia*, 11.3 (1996): 47-70.

Nagel, M. "Reviewed Works: Motherhood Lost by Linda Layne" *NWSE Journal*, 16.3 (2004): 233-235.

Neugebauer, R., et al. "Determinants of depressive symptoms in the early weeks after miscarriage." *American Journal of Public Health*, 82.10 (1992): 1332-1339.

Parsons, K. "Feminist reflections on miscarriage, in light of abortion. *Int. Journal of Feminist Approaches to Bioethics*, 3.1 (2010): 1-22.

Reagan, L. "From hazard to blessing to tragedy: representations of miscarriage in twentieth century America." *Feminist Studies* 29.2 (2003): 356-378.

Reinharz, S. "What's missing in miscarriage?" *Journal of Community Psychology*, 16.1 (1988): 84-103.

Swanson, K., et al. "Contexts and evolution of women's responses to miscarriage during the first year after loss." *Research in Nursing and Health* 30 (2007): 2-16.

Taylor, J. "Confronting 'culture' in medicine's 'culture of no culture'." *Academic Medicine*, 78.6 (2003): 555-559.

Wolf, N. *Misconceptions: Truth, Lies, and the Unexpected on the Journey to Motherhood*. New York: Doubleday, 2001. Print.

www.ingramcontent.com/pod-product-compliance
Lightning Source LLC
Chambersburg PA
CBHW070151290526
45789CB00002B/717